KETO DIET AFTER 50:

Reduce Your Weight While Eating the Food You Love. A Guide to Ketogenic Diet for Senior with a 28-Day Meal Plan to Reset Your Metabolism and stay Healthy.

AMY CONTESSA

© Copyright 2020 - All rights reserved.

The content contained within this book may not be reproduced, duplicated or transmitted without direct written permission from the author or the publisher. Under no circumstances will any blame or legal responsibility be held against the publisher, or author, for any damages, reparation, or monetary loss due to the information contained within this book. Either directly or indirectly.

Legal Notice:

This book is copyright protected. This book is only for personal use. You cannot amend, distribute, sell, use, quote or paraphrase any part, or the content within this book, without the consent of the author or publisher.

Disclaimer Notice:

Please note the information contained within this document is for educational and entertainment purposes only. All effort has been executed to present accurate, up to date, and reliable, complete information. No warranties of any kind are declared or implied. Readers acknowledge that the author is not engaging in the rendering of legal, financial, medical or professional advice. The content within this book has been derived from various sources. Please consult a licensed professional before attempting any techniques outlined in this book.

By reading this document, the reader agrees that under no circumstances is the author responsible for any losses, direct or indirect, which are incurred as a result of the use of information contained within this document, including, but not limited to, errors, omissions, or inaccuracies.

TABLE OF CONTENTS

INTRODUCTION 6

CHAPTER 1: THE KETO DIET BASICS 8
- Types of Keto Diet 8
- The Standard Ketogenic Diet (SKD): 8
- Targeted Ketogenic Diet (TKD) 8
- High-Protein Ketogenic Diet 8
- Recurring Ketogenic Diet (RKD) 9
- Very Low Carbs Ketogenic Diet (VLCKD) 9
- The MCTs Ketogenic Diet: 9
- The Calorie Restricted Ketogenic Diet 9
- Signs and Symptoms, You're in Ketosis 10

CHAPTER 2: CALORIES AND NUTRITION 12

CHAPTER 3: GETTING STARTED ON KETO AFTER 50 14
- Seafood 14
- Low-carb Vegetables 14
- Fruits Low in Sugar 14
- Meat and Eggs 15
- Nuts and Seeds 15
- Dairy Products 15
- Oils 15
- Coffee and Tea 16
- Dark Chocolate 16
- Sugar Substitutes 16
- Foods to Avoid 17
- Bread and Grains 17
- Fruits 17
- Vegetables 17
- Pasta 17
- Cereal 18

CHAPTER 4: BREAKFAST RECIPES 20
- French Omelet 20
- Sage Sausage Patty 21
- Feta Frittata 22
- Ham Steak With Bacon, Mushrooms, and Gruyere 23
- Mushroom-Mascarpone Frittata 24
- Broccoli Quiche Cups 25
- Savory Chicken Sausage-Apple 26
- Manchego and Shiitake Scramble 27
- Three-Cheese Quiche 28
- Breakfast Turkey Sausage 29
- No-Bread Breakfast Sandwich 30
- Baked Eggs 31
- Cured Salmon With Chives and Scrambled Eggs..32
- Eggs Benedict on Avocados 33

CHAPTER 5: SEAFOOD / FISH 34
- Keto Baked Salmon with Lemon and Butter 34
- Ketogenic Spicy Oyster 35
- Garlic Lime Mahi-Mahi 36
- Fish and Leek Sauté 37
- Smoked Salmon Salad 38
- Keto Baked Salmon with Pesto 39
- Roasted Salmon with Parmesan Dill Crust 40
- Keto Fried Salmon with Broccoli and Cheese 41

CHAPTER 6: BEEF, LAMB AND PORK 42
- Herbed Beef Tenderloin 42
- Steak with Cheese Sauce 43
- Steak with Pesto 45
- Herbed Lamb Chops 46
- Stuffed Leg of Lamb 47
- Grilled Pork Chops 48
- Pork Chops in Cream Sauce 49
- Sweet & Tangy Pork Tenderloin 50

CHAPTER 7: POULTRY RECIPES 52
- Grilled Whole Chicken 52
- Grilled Chicken Breast 53
- Glazed Chicken Thighs 54
- Bacon-Wrapped Chicken Breasts 55
- Chicken Parmigiana 57
- Roasted Turkey 59
- Roasted Turkey Breast 61

CHAPTER 8: SALAD RECIPES 62

    Roasted Brussels Sprouts Salad with Parmesan . 63
    Wedge Salad 64
    Mexican Egg Salad 65
    Blue Cheese and Bacon Kale Salad 66
    Chopped Greek Salad 67
    Mediterranean Cucumber Salad 68
    Avocado Egg Salad Lettuce Cups 69

CHAPTER 9: VEGETABLES 70

    Avocado Chips 70
    Parmesan Zucchini Fries 71
    Tofu with Peanut Dipping Sauce 72
    Cream Cheese Mini Multi Sweet Peppers 73
    Corn On the Cob 74
    Corn Nuts 75
    Toasted Broccoli and Cauliflower 76
    Air Fried, Roasted Okra 77
    Vegetable Pakoras 78
    Cauliflower Rice 79
    Keto Mushroom Soup 80
    Broccoli Salmon 81

CHAPTER 10: SOUP RECIPES 82

    Creamy Broccoli and Leek Soup 82
    Chicken Soup 83
    Greek Egg and Lemon Soup with Chicken 84
    Wild Mushroom Soup 85
    Roasted Butternut Squash Soup 86
    Zucchini Cream Soup 87
    Cauli Soup 88
    Thai Coconut Soup 89
    Chicken Ramen Soup 90
    Egg Drop Soup 91

CHAPTER 11: DESSERT 92

    Sugar-Free Lemon Bars 92
    Creamy Hot Chocolate 93
    Delicious Coffee Ice Cream 94
    Fatty Bombs with Cinnamon and Cardamom 95
    Raspberry Mousse 96
    Chocolate Spread with Hazelnuts 97
    Quick and Simple Brownie 98
    Cute Peanut Balls 99
    Chocolate Mug Muffins 100

CHAPTER 12: 28-DAY KETO MEAL PLAN FOR PEOPLE OVER 50 102

CHAPTER 13: COMMON MISTAKES IN THE KETOGENIC DIET YOU NEED TO KNOW 106

    Benefits of The Keto Diet for People Over 50 109
    Keto Side Effects and How to Salve Them 110

CONCLUSION 114

Introduction

Most people try the keto diet to lose weight and for good reasons too. It is more effective than a traditional low-fat diet. There is also solid evidence that shows that the diet reduces seizures in children. Research proves it can prevent or provide relief from the symptoms of brain disorders like Alzheimer's, Parkinson's, autism, multiple sclerosis, sleep disorders, and even brain cancer. The ketogenic diet provides better blood sugar control and improves the level of cholesterol. There are other benefits too.

It works for everyone… both children and people over 50. There is data on children who have been eating the keto prescribed foods for more than 12 years without any side effects. There is also evidence that shows that the diet is safe for seniors. But remember, the diet cannot be a replacement for a doctor.

There are a few side effects, but they are not very serious. For instance, when you first start the diet, you can have the 'keto flu' because your body is still getting accustomed to eating fewer carbohydrates. There can also be nausea, headaches, muscle cramps, fogginess, and fatigue. These symptoms will not last for more than a week.

In the meantime, make sure to get enough sleep. Stay properly hydrated.

The 'basal metabolic rate', which is the number of calories required every day for survival, goes down with advancing age. However, the seniors will still require the same amount of nutrients as younger people. When you follow the ketogenic diet, your body will receive a lot of nutrition per calorie, making the keto diet an excellent choice.

Also remember, people over 50 years of age will face more problems if they eat too many junk foods. That's because the body will not be so resilient like the younger days. So it is critical that the seniors eat foods that support their health and can help them fight diseases. It can make the crucial difference between enjoying their golden years or spending time in agony and pain.

So the seniors must opt for an optimal diet and avoid empty calories from sugar or from foods that have anti-nutrients like wholegrains. They must consume more proteins and nutrient-rich fats. But sadly, the seniors will often eat too many processed foods and those with poor nutrients like pasta, white bread, mashed potatoes, prunes, puddings, and such others. This can cause poor health.

High carbohydrate diets are not good for the long-term health of those who are more than 50 years of age. It is best to switch to a low-carb diet that offers plant and animal fats. It promotes better insulin sensitivity, reduces cognitive decline, and improves health overall.

We must always eat healthy foods so that we can feel and function at our best, no matter what the age. It is, of course, even more, important that people over 50 eat healthy foods because the body's strength and disease-fighting abilities will go down with time. But it is never too late to start. The sooner you start, the better will be your chance to avoid diseases. Ketosis can even repair damages caused by years of neglect or eating unhealthy food.

Remember, health problems will become more serious with age. So eat foods that will help you maintain a healthy weight, improve your immunity, let you control the blood sugar levels, provide vital nutrients, and control the cholesterol level.

To lead a long and healthy life, we must make the right decisions today. Unhealthy choices can cause pain and suffering later.

CHAPTER 1:

The Keto Diet Basics

Types of Keto Diet

There are several types of Ketogenic diet that you could adapt and maintain. These include;

The Standard Ketogenic Diet (SKD):

In simple terms, this is a very low-carb diet accompanied by high-fats and moderate protein that is consumed by human beings. It consists of 70% to 75% fats, 20% protein and about 5% to 10% carbs. This translates to about 20 – 45 grams of carbohydrates, 40 – 65 grams of proteins, but no set limits for fats, which makes up for large parts of the diet. This is because fats are what provide the calories which constitute energy and make the diet a successful Ketogenic diet. Additionally, there is no limit to the fats because different human beings have different energy requirements. The Standard Ketogenic Diet is successful in assisting people in losing weight, improving the body's glucose as well as improving heart health.

Targeted Ketogenic Diet (Tkd)

This type of Ketogenic Diet focuses its attention on the addition of carbs during workout sessions only. This type of Ketogenic diet is almost similar to the Standard Ketogenic Diet except for the fact that carbohydrates are all but consumed during workout sessions. This type of diet is solely based on the idea that the body will effectively and efficiently process carbohydrates consumed before or during a workout session. This is because the diet assumes that the muscles would be bound to demand more energy, which would be provided by the carbohydrates consumed and be processed quickly since the body is in an active state. This diet, in simpler terms, is a diet caught up between the Cyclical Ketogenic diet and the Standard Ketogenic Diet, which allows room for consumption of carbohydrates on the days that you would decide to work out only.

High-Protein Ketogenic Diet

This type of Ketogenic Diet advocates for more protein compared to the Standard Ketogenic Diet. This diet consists of 35% protein, 60% fats, and 5% carbs, unlike the Standard Ketogenic Diet. Research has dramatically suggested that this diet would be useful for you if you are attempting to lose weight. However, unlike other types of the Ketogenic diet, no research has been dedicated to showing if there are any side effects of adapting to the diet for elongated periods.

Recurring Ketogenic Diet (RKD)

This kind of Ketogenic Diet focuses on higher-carb re-feeds, for instance, 5 Ketogenic days and two high-carb days, and this cycle is repeated. This diet is also known as the carb backloading. It is often intended for athletes because the diet allows their bodies to recover the glycogen lost as a result of workouts or intense sporting activities.

Very Low Carbs Ketogenic Diet (VLCKD)

As stated, prior, a Ketogenic diet will most likely consist of very low carbs; thus, this diet often refers to the characteristics of the Standard Ketogenic Diet.

The Well Formulated Ketogenic Diet:

this term is as a result of one of the leading researchers into the Ketogenic diet, Steve Phinney. As the name suggests, this diet has its fats, carbohydrates, and proteins well-formulated, and that it meets the standards of a Ketogenic diet. This diet is also similar to the Standard Ketogenic Diet, and this means that it creates room for your body to undergo Ketosis effectively.

The MCTs Ketogenic Diet:

The diet is also related to the Standard Ketogenic Diet only that it derives most of its fats from medium-chain triglycerides (MCTs). This diet will often use coconut oil, which has high levels of MCTs. This diet has been reported to efficiently treat epilepsy because of its concept that MCTs give your body enough room to consume carbohydrates as well as proteins and still maintain your body's Ketosis. This is a result of MCTs providing more ketones per gram in fat, contrary to the long-chain triglycerides, which are more common in the average dietary fats. However, MCTs could lead to diarrhea as well as stomach upsets if this diet is consumed in large quantities on its own. To handle, it is wise to prepare a meal with a balance of both MCTs and fats with no MCTs. There is no evidence to prove that this diet could as well have benefits in your attempt to losing weight or if the diet could regulate your body's blood sugar.

The Calorie Restricted Ketogenic Diet

This is also related to the Standard Ketogenic Diet except that its calories are only limited to a given amount. Research has proven that Ketogenic diets could be successful whether the consumption of calories is restricted or not. The reason behind this is that the effect of consuming fats and your body being in Ketosis is a way in itself that prevents you from over-eating or eating beyond your limits. There are numerous Ketogenic diets, but the Standard Ketogenic Diet and the High-Protein Ketogenic Diets are the most studied and most recommended for health issues. The Repeated (cyclical) and Targeted Ketogenic diets remain mostly practiced by athletes and bodybuilders and are more advanced than the Standard Ketogenic Diet and the High-Protein Ketogenic Diet. Visit and consult your local physician before opting to settle on any of the types of Ketogenic diets.

Signs and Symptoms, You're in Ketosis

As you practice the ketogenic diet further, you will be able to tell you are in Ketosis through the signs and symptoms you are going to experience. Remember that you will now be providing your body with a new fuel source. It is going to take a little bit of time to adapt your body to this change. Below, you will find the most common symptoms of Ketosis to tell if you are following the diet correctly.

Bad Breath

I know, a great introduction to the ketogenic diet, but bad breath is one of the most reported symptoms for individuals who have reached full Ketosis. The good news is that this is a widespread side effect for individuals who follow a low-carb diet. Some have described the scent as a "fruit" smell.

Elevated ketone levels in your body cause this scent. The smell is the acetone that exits your body through breath and urine. And while this symptom is less than ideal for your friends and family, it is an excellent sign that you are following your diet correctly! To solve this issue, you will want to brush your teeth a few times a day or find a sugar-free gum to chew on.

Increased Ketones in Blood, Urine, or Breath

As mentioned earlier, you will want to find a way of testing ketones in your body. One of the best ways to do this is to test your blood ketone levels using a meter. When you do this, the meter will be able to measure the amount of BHB in your blood, one of the primary ketones that will be present in your bloodstream. If you are in true Ketosis, your blood ketones should be anywhere from .5-3.0 mmol/L.

Weight Loss

When you first begin the ketogenic diet, weight loss can happen almost immediately. Some have reported that weight loss has even occurred in the first week! If this happens, the weight loss is most likely coming from the water and carbs that have been stored in your body. After the initial drop in weight, you should expect to lose body fat consistently. It will be up to you to stick to the diet to keep the weight loss up!

Decreased Appetite

Another common symptom of the ketogenic diet is appetite suppression. Many individuals have reported that while following this diet, they aren't as hungry as they used to be. Potentially, this could be due to the increased protein intake and alterations to the hunger hormones through Ketosis. Either way, a decreased appetite means increased weight loss. It is a win-win situation for anyone following the ketogenic diet.

Increased Energy

When your body enters Ketosis, you will probably experience a new boost of energy that you didn't even know you had in you! Of course, increased energy and focus are a long-term effect of the diet. When you first start, you will most likely experience symptoms such as tiredness and brain fog. Fret not, as this is to be expected as your body adapts to a new fuel source.

The good news is that once you are in Ketosis, your brain is going to start burning these ketones instead of glucose. This is a very potent fuel for your mind, which is why followers of this diet have <u>reported</u> improved brain function and clarity.

Fatigue

As mentioned earlier, more than likely, you will experience some fatigue if you are just getting started on the ketogenic diet. On top of exhaustion, you may feel overall weak, which is a pretty common side effect of the ketogenic diet. As you probably realize, the switch to running on ketones isn't going to happen overnight. Instead, you should expect these symptoms to subside anywhere from seven to thirty days. To help combat the fatigue, consider taking an electrolyte supplement.

Digestive Issues

Another common symptom of starting this diet is experiencing digestive issues. When you make such a drastic change to your diet, it involves changing the types of foods you eat daily. When this happens, digestive problems like diarrhea and constipation are to be expected. While these symptoms will subside, you may want to take note of which foods you feel are causing these issues...

CHAPTER 2:

Calories And Nutrition

Your food intake for the day should be as clean as possible because this can help you to get a youthful look. Consider looking into whole foods diets such as Paleo, Juicing, or Plant-Strong, since these are simple to follow and will give you the basics of how to cut out processed and toxin-filled junk. Most of these diets are not expensive despite what you may think and you might actually find yourself saving money as well as losing weight. Whole foods are good because they're often much more filling than junk and because they're rich in all the anti-aging nutrients you could possibly need. In fact, if you're using a food tracker, simply eating cleaner may mean you won't even need a multivitamin or some anti-aging supplements (like high-dose Vitamin C). If at all possible, get your nutrients from your food, they're better quality and much easier for the body to absorb than the pharmaceutical versions. Remember that calorie restriction is important when it comes to eating well for anti-aging.

At the end of your day, head home to another nutritious meal, but don't forget to spend time with people that you care about. Being present in your life will make it much more meaningful, what's the point in living 100 years if you don't enjoy it? By being social and present, you'll also get the anti-aging benefits of doing so as well as create better memories for yourself. Consider getting together to do something active as you'll need to be up and moving at least 30 minutes a day. If you haven't yet done your yoga consider looking into partner-yoga or classes together. Partner yoga is an ideal way to bring you closer together too. If possible, try to do this in places of nature. Being around nature has been proven to have a positive impact on the brain.

If you're going to head to the gym, try and find one that has a sauna. The reason for this is that sweating is one of the most efficient ways for your body to get rid of toxins. Cigarette smoke and sun damage can all age your skin through toxins, but these are quickly sweated out in a sauna. Studies have shown that by using a sauna regularly, you can help reduce the appearance of wrinkles temporarily. As the steam penetrates the skin, the pores open up, releasing anything in the cells to the steam. You'll only need to spend 10-20 minutes in there to feel the beneficial effects.

Don't forget your supplement regime throughout the day. Many anti-aging supplements need to be taken at specific times or with meals, so plan your supplements accordingly and consider getting a pill organizer if you can't remember them.

When you finally head to bed, you'll want to make sure that you're moisturizing your skin again. If you didn't make your eight glasses of water, consider having one before bed to top up what you've missed. A hot cup of tea is also an ideal way to relax before bed. Lavender oil has many anti-aging properties and is also great for relaxation. You can take lavender as a relaxing tea before bed or put a few drops of the oil onto your pillow before going to bed.

The key to being successful in this plan is that you need to be able to fit as many of these things into your daily routine as possible. It's fairly established that if you can do something for seven days, then it will become a hàbit, so simply trying to do it for that long before saying you can't is important. But, above all, if you didn't make your eight glasses, haven't done your yoga, or ate that hamburger – Don't stress about it! A little slip now and then happens, so let it go and remember that tomorrow is another day.

CHAPTER 3:

Getting Started On Keto After 50

I've had people complain about the difficulty of switching their grocery list to one that's Ketogenic-friendly. The fact is that food is expensive – and most of the food you have in your fridge is probably packed full of carbohydrates. This is why if you're committing to a Ketogenic Diet, you need to do a clean sweep. That's right – everything that's packed with carbohydrates should be identified and set aside to make sure you're not eating more than you should. You can donate them to a charity before going out and buying your new Keto-friendly shopping list.

Seafood

Seafood means fish like sardines, mackerel, and wild salmon. It's also a good idea to add some shrimp, tuna, mussels, and crab into your diet. This is going to be a tad expensive, but worth it in the long run. What's the common denominator in all these food items? The secret is omega-3 fatty acids, which are credited for lots of health benefits. You want to add food rich in omega-3 fatty acids to your diet.

Low-carb Vegetables

Not all vegetables are good for you when it comes to the Ketogenic Diet. The vegetable choices should be limited to those with low carbohydrate counts. Pack up your cart with items like spinach, eggplant, arugula, broccoli, and cauliflower. You can also put in bell peppers, cabbage, celery, kale, Brussels sprouts, mushrooms, zucchini, and fennel. So what's in them? Well, aside from the fact that they're low-carb, these vegetables also contain loads of fiber, which makes digestion easier. Of course, there's also the presence of vitamins, minerals, antioxidants, and various other nutrients that you need for day to day life. Which ones should you avoid? Steer clear of the starch-packed vegetables like carrots, turnips, and beets. As a rule, you go for the vegetables that are green and leafy.

Fruits Low in Sugar

During an episode of sugar-craving, it's usually a good idea to pick low-sugar fruit items. Believe it or not, there are lots of those in the market! Just make sure to stock up on any of these: avocado, blackberries, raspberries, strawberries, blueberries, lime, lemon, and coconut. Also, note that tomatoes are fruits too, so feel free to make side dishes or dips with loads of tomatoes! Keep in mind that these fruits should be eaten fresh and not out of a can.

If you do eat them fresh off the can, however, take a good look at the nutritional information at the back of the packaging. Avocadoes are particularly popular for those practicing the Ketogenic Diet because they contain LOTS of the good kind of fat.

Meat and Eggs

While some diets will tell you to skip the meat, the Ketogenic Diet encourages its consumption. Meat is packed with protein that will feed your muscles and give you a consistent source of energy throughout the day. It's a slow but sure burn when you eat protein as opposed to carbohydrates, which are burned faster and therefore stored faster if you don't use them immediately.

But what kind of meat should you be eating? There's chicken, beef, pork, venison, turkey, and lamb. Keep in mind that quality plays a huge role here – you should be eating grass-fed organic beef or organic poultry if you want to make the most out of this food variety. The nuclear option lets you limit the possibility of ingesting toxins in your body due to the production process of these products. Plus, the preservation process also means there are added salt or sugar in the meat, which can throw off the whole diet.

Nuts and Seeds

Nuts and seeds you should add to your cart include chia seeds, brazil nuts, macadamia nuts, flaxseed, walnuts, hemp seeds, pecans, sesame seeds, almonds, hazelnut, and pumpkin seeds. They also contain lots of protein and very little sugar, so they're great if you have the munchies. They're the ideal snack because they're quick, easy, and will keep you full. They're high in calories, though, which is why lots of people steer clear of them. As I mentioned earlier, though – the Ketogenic Diet has nothing to do with calories and everything to do with the nutrient you're eating. So don't pay too much attention to the calorie count and just remember that they're a good source of fats and protein.

Dairy Products

OK – some people in their 50s already have a hard time processing dairy products, but for those who don't – you can happily add many of these to your diet. Make sure to consume sufficient amounts of cheese, plain Greek yogurt, cream butter, and cottage cheese. These dairy products are packed with calcium, protein, and a healthy kind of fat.

Oils

Nope, we're not talking about essentials oils but rather MCT oil, coconut oil, avocado oil, nut oils, and even extra-virgin olive oil. You can start using those for your frying needs to create healthier food options. The beauty of these oils is that they add flavor to the food, making sure you don't get bored quickly with the recipes. Try picking up different types of Keto-friendly oils to add some variety to your cooking.

Coffee and Tea

The good news is that you don't have to skip coffee if you're going on a Ketogenic Diet. The bad news is that you can't go to Starbucks anymore and order their blended coffee choices. Instead, beverages would be limited to unsweetened tea or unsweetened coffee to keep sugar consumption low. Opt for organic coffee and tea products to make the most out of these powerful antioxidants.

Dark Chocolate

Yes – chocolate is still on the menu, but it is limited to just dark chocolate. Technically, this means eating chocolate that is 70 percent cacao, which would make the taste a bit bitter.

Sugar Substitutes

While sweeteners are an important part of food preparation, you can't just use any kind of sugar in your recipe. Remember: the regular sugar is pure carbohydrate. Even if you're not eating carbohydrates, if you're dumping lots of sugar in your food – you're not following the Ketogenic Diet principles.

So what do you do? You find sugar substitutes. The good news is that there are LOTS of those in the market. You can get rid of the old sugar and use any of these as a good substitute.

Stevia: This is perhaps the most familiar one in this list. It's a natural sweetener derived from plants and contains very few calories. Unlike your regular sugar, stevia may help lower the sugar levels instead of causing it to spike. Note, though, that it's sweeter than actual sugar, so when cooking with stevia, you'll need to lower the amount used. Typically, the ratio is 200 grams of sugar per 1 teaspoon of powdered stevia.

Sucralose: It contains zero calories and zero carbohydrates. It's an artificial sweetener and does not metabolize – hence the complete lack of carbohydrates. Splenda is a sweetener derived from sucralose. Note, though, that you don't want to use this as a baking substitute for sugar. Its best use is for coffee, yogurt, and oatmeal sweetening. Note though that like stevia, it's also very sweet, it's actually 600 times sweeter than the regular sugar. Use sparingly.

Erythritol: It's a naturally occurring compound that interacts with the tongue's sweet taste receptors. Hence, it mimics the taste of sugar without actually being sugar. It does contain calories, but only about 5% of the calories you'll find in the regular sugar. Note, though, that it doesn't dissolve very well, so anything prepared with this sweetener will have a gritty feeling. This can be problematic if you're using the product for baking. As for sweetness, the typical ratio is 1 1/3 cup for 1 cup of sugar.

Xylitol: Like erythritol, xylitol is a type of sugar alcohol that's commonly used in sugar-free gum. While it still contains calories, the calories are just 3 per gram. It's a sweetener that's good for diabetic patients because it doesn't raise the sugar levels of insulin in the body. The great thing about this is that you don't have to do any computations when using it for baking, cooking, or fixing a drink. The ratio of it with sugar is 1 to 1, so you can quickly make the substitution in the recipe.

Foods to Avoid
Bread and Grains

Bread is a staple food in many countries. You have loaves, bagels, tortillas, and the list goes on. However, no matter what form bread takes, they still pack a lot of carbs. The same applies to whole-grain as well because they are made from refined flour.

Depending on your daily carb limit, eating a sandwich or bagel can put your way over your daily limit. So if you really want to eat bread, it is best to make keto variants at home instead.

Grains such as rice, wheat, and oats pack a lot of carbs as well. So limit or avoid that as well.

Fruits

Fruits are healthy for you. In fact, they have been linked to a lower risk of heart disease and cancer. However, there are a few that you need to avoid in your keto diets. The problem is that some of those foods pack quite a lot of carbs such as banana, raisins, dates, mango, and pear.

As a general rule, avoid sweet and dried fruits. Berries are an exception because they do not contain as much sugar and are rich in fiber. So you can still eat some of them, around 50 grams. Moderation is key.

Vegetables

Vegetables are just as healthy for your body. Most of the keto diet does not care how many vegetables you eat so long as they are low in starch. Vegetables that are rich in fiber can help with weight loss. For one, they make you feel full for longer so they help suppress your appetite. Another benefit is that your body would burn more calories to break and digest them. Moreover, they help control blood sugar and aid with your bowel movements.

But that also means you need to avoid or limit vegetables that are high in starch because they have more carbs than fiber. That includes corn, potato, sweet potato, and beets.

Pasta

Pasta is also a staple food in many countries. It is versatile and convenient. As with any other convenient food, pasta is rich in carbs. So when you are on your keto diet, spaghetti or any other types of pasta are not recommended. You can probably get away with it by eating a small portion, but that is not possible.

Thankfully, that does not mean you need to give up on it altogether. If you are craving pasta, you can try some other alternatives that are low in carbs such as spiralized veggies or shirataki noodles.

Cereal

Cereal is also a huge offender because sugary breakfast cereals pack a lot of carbs. That also applies to "healthy cereals." Just because they use other words to describe their product does not mean that you should believe them. That also applies to oatmeal, whole-grain cereals, etc.

So when you eat a bowl of cereal when you are doing keto, you are already way over your carb limit, and we haven't even added milk into the equation! Therefore, avoid whole-grain cereal or cereals that we mention here altogether.

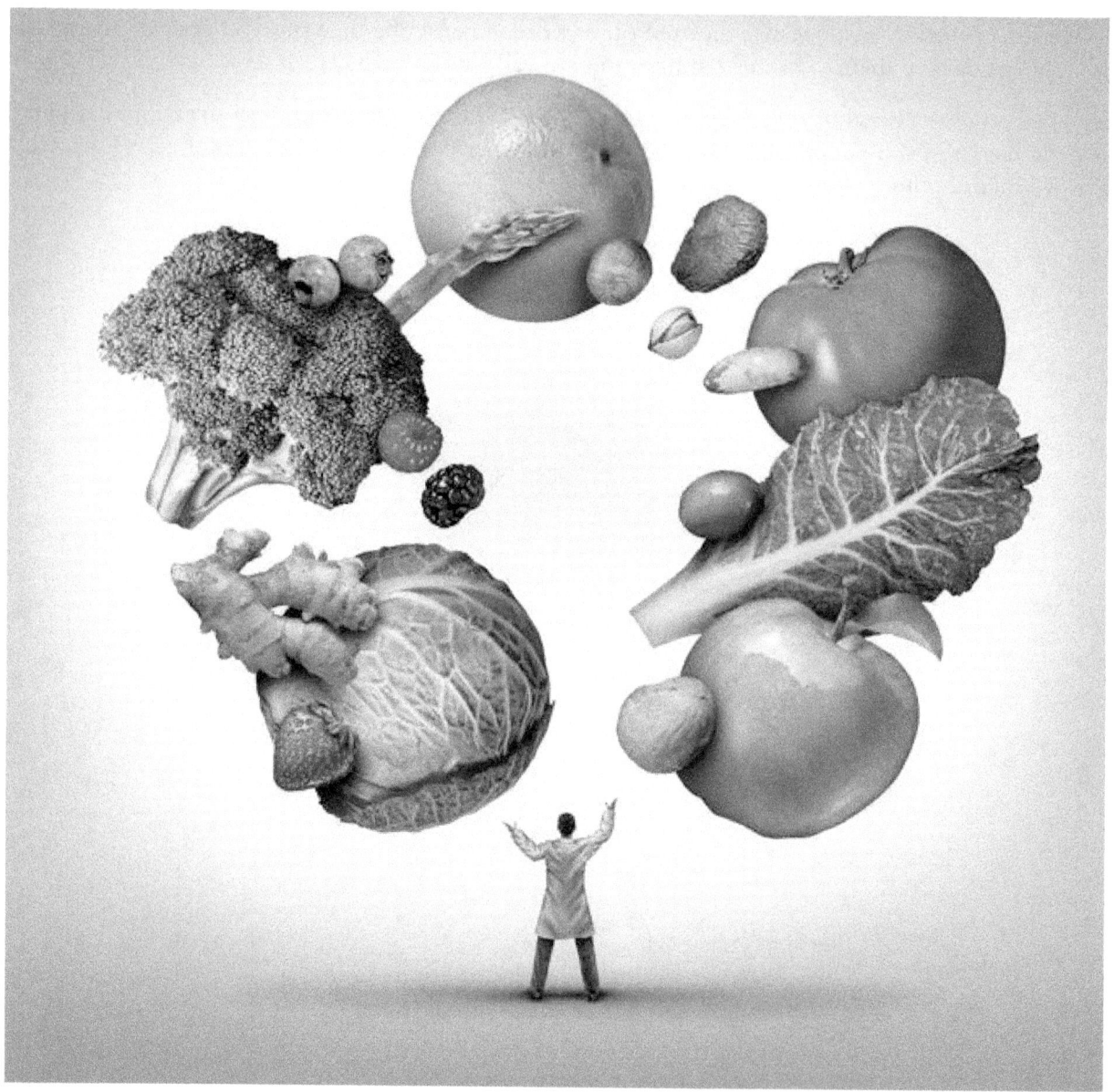

CHAPTER 4:

Breakfast Recipes

French Omelet

Preparation Time: Twenty minutes

Cooking Time: Two servings

Ingredients

Two large eggs

Four egg whites

One-fourth cup of milk

One-eighth tsp. of each

Pepper

Salt

One cup of ham (cooked)

One tbsp. of each

Green pepper (chopped)

Onion (chopped)

Half cup of cheddar cheese (shredded)

Directions:

Whisk the first five listed ingredients. Use cooking spray for greasing a skillet. Place the skillet over medium flame. Add the mixture of eggs. Cook for two minutes. Top with the remaining ingredients. Fold the egg in half. Cut the omelet in half. Serve immediately.

Nutrition:

Calories: 189 Protein: 22.3g Carbs: 3.6gFat: 10.9g Fiber: 0.1g

Sage Sausage Patty

Preparation Time: One hour and fifteen minutes

Cooking Time: Thirty minutes

Servings: Eight servings

Ingredients

One pound of pork (ground)

Three-fourth cup of cheddar cheese (ground)

One-fourth cup of buttermilk

One tbsp. of onion (chopped)

Two tsps. of sage

Three-fourth tsp. of each

Pepper

Salt

Half tsp. of each

Oregano (dried)

Garlic powder

Directions:

Combine the listed ingredients either in a bowl or in a food processor.

Shape the mixture into eight equal patties of half-inch. Refrigerate the patties for one hour.

Heat oil in an iron skillet. Cook the patties on each side for six minutes.

Serve hot.

Nutrition:

Calories: 160.3 Protein: 14.6g Carbs: 1.2gFat: 12.3g Fiber: 0.3g

Feta Frittata

Preparation Time: Thirty minutes

Cooking Time: Thirty minutes

Servings: Two servings

Ingredients

One green onion (sliced)

One clove of garlic (minced)

Two large eggs

Half cup of egg substitute

Four tbsps. of feta cheese (crumbled)

One-third cup of plum tomato (chopped)

Four slices of avocado (peeled)

Two tbsps. of sour cream

Directions:

Heat oil in an iron skillet. Add garlic and onion. Sauté for three minutes.

Combine egg substitute, eggs, and three tbsps. of feta cheese in a bowl. Add the mixture of eggs to the skillet.

Cook for six minutes.

Sprinkle remaining feta and tomato from the top.

Cover and cook for two minutes.

Let the egg stand for five minutes.

Serve with sour cream and avocado.

Nutrition:

Calories: 205.3 Protein: 19.3g Carbs: 6.7gFat: 12.5g Fiber: 3.6g

Ham Steak With Bacon, Mushrooms, and Gruyere

Preparation Time: Thirty-five minutes

Cooking Time: Thirty minutes

Servings: Four servings

Ingredients

Two tbsps. of butter

Half pound of mushrooms (sliced)

One shallot (chopped)

Two cloves of garlic (minced)

One-eighth tsp. of black pepper (ground)

One boneless ham steak (cooked, cut in four equal pieces)

One cup of gruyere cheese (shredded)

Four strips of bacon (cooked, crumbled)

One tbsp. of parsley (minced)

Directions:

Heat butter in a large iron skillet. Add shallot and mushrooms. Cook the mixture for six minutes. Mix garlic and pepper. Sauté for two minutes. Keep aside.

Cook the ham in the same skillet. Add bacon and cheese. Cook for two minutes.

Serve the ham with the mushroom mixture from the top.

Nutrition:

Calories: 356.3 Protein: 35.4g Carbs: 5.1gFat: 23.2g Fiber: 1.1g

Mushroom-Mascarpone Frittata

Preparation Time: Forty-five minutes

Cooking Time: Thirty minutes

Servings: Six servings

Ingredients

Eight large eggs

One-third cup of whipping cream

Half cup of Romano cheese (grated)

Two tsps. of salt

Five tbsps. of olive oil

Three-fourth pound of fresh mushrooms (sliced)

One onion (sliced)

Two tbsps. of basil (minced)

Two cloves of garlic (minced)

One-eighth tsp. of pepper

Eight ounces of mascarpone cheese

Directions:

Whisk together cream, eggs, one-fourth cup of Romano cheese, and salt in a bowl.

Heat two tbsps. of oil in a pan. Add mushrooms and onion. Sauté for two minutes. Add garlic, basil, along with pepper. Stir for one minute. Remove from heat. Add Romano cheese and mascarpone cheese. Heat one tbsp. of oil in the same pan. Add half mixture of eggs in the pan. Keep cooking for seven minutes. Repeat with the remaining egg mixture.

Place one egg frittata on a plate. Add the mixture of mushrooms. Spread properly.

Add the other layer of frittata.

Cut in wedges. Serve immediately.

Nutrition:

Calories: 469.3 Protein: 18.7g Carbs: 5.7gFat: 45.4g Fiber: 1.6g

Broccoli Quiche Cups

Preparation Time: Twenty-five minutes

Cooking Time: Thirty minutes

Servings: Six servings

Ingredients

One cup of broccoli (chopped)

One and a half cup of pepper jack cheese (shredded)

Six large eggs

Three-fourth cup of whipping cream

Half cup of bacon bits

One shallot (minced)

One-fourth tsp. of each

Pepper

Salt

Directions:

Preheat your oven at one-hundred and seventy degrees Celsius.

Divide the cheese and chopped broccoli among twelve greased muffin cups.

Combine the remaining ingredients in a bowl. Divide the prepared mixture among the cups.

Bake the quiche cups for twenty minutes.

Serve immediately.

Nutrition:

Calories: 292.3 Protein: 17.6g Carbs: 3.6gFat: 25.4g Fiber: 0.7g

Savory Chicken Sausage-Apple

Preparation Time: Twenty-five minutes

Cooking Time: Thirty minutes

Servings: Four servings

Ingredients

One tart apple (peeled, diced)

Two tsps. of poultry seasoning

One tsp. of salt

One-fourth tsp. of pepper

One pound of chicken (ground)

Directions:

Take a large bowl. Mix the first four ingredients. Crumble the chicken over the apple mixture. Combine well. Shape the mixture into eight equal patties of three-inch.

Heat oil in an iron skillet.

Cook the apple-chicken patties for six minutes on each side.

Serve hot.

Nutrition:

Calories: 93.6 Protein: 9.9g Carbs: 3.2gFat: 6.5g Fiber: 1.2g

Manchego and Shiitake Scramble

Preparation Time: Twenty-five minutes

Cooking Time: Thirty minutes

Servings: Eight servings

Ingredients

Two tbsps. of olive oil

Half cup of each

Sweet red pepper (diced)

Onion (diced)

Two cups of shiitake mushrooms (sliced)

One tsp. of prepared horseradish

Eight large eggs (beaten)

One cup of each

Whipping cream

Manchego cheese (shredded)

Half tsp. of each

Pepper (ground)

Kosher salt

Directions:

Heat one tbsp. of oil in an iron skillet. Add red pepper and onion. Cook for three minutes. Cook the mixture for four minutes after adding the mushrooms along with horseradish. Stir for two minutes.

Whisk the remaining ingredients in a bowl with some olive oil. Pour the mixture into the skillet.

Cook and scramble the eggs for four minutes.

Serve hot.

Nutrition:

Calories: 270.6 Protein: 12.1g Carbs: 3.4gFat: 23.6g Fiber: 1.1g

Three-Cheese Quiche

Preparation Time: One hour and ten minutes

Cooking Time: Thirty minutes

Servings: Six servings

Ingredients

Seven large eggs

Five egg yolks

One cup of each

Whipping cream

Half and half cream

Mozzarella cheese (shredded)

Three-fourth cup of cheddar cheese (shredded)

Half cup of Swiss cheese (shredded)

Two tbsps. of sun-dried tomatoes

One and half tsp. of seasoning blend

One-fourth tsp. of basil (dried)

Directions:

Preheat your oven at one hundred and fifty degrees Celsius.

Combine egg yolks, eggs, whipping cream, mozzarella cheese, half and half cream, half cup of cheddar cheese, tomatoes, Swiss cheese, basil, and seasoning blend in a greased pie dish. Sprinkle the remaining cheddar cheese from the top.

Bake for fifty minutes.

Let the quiche sit for ten minutes.

Cut in triangles and serve.

Nutrition:

Calories: 448.3 Protein: 21.2g Carbs: 5.2gFat: 38.6g Fiber: 0.2g

Breakfast Turkey Sausage

Preparation Time: Twenty minutes

Cooking Time: Thirty minutes

Servings: Eight servings

Ingredients

One pound of lean turkey (ground)

Three-fourth tsp. of salt

Half tsp. of rubbed sage

One-fourth tsp. of ginger (ground)

One-third tsp. of pepper (ground)

Directions:

Crumble the turkey meat in a large bowl. Add sage, salt, ginger, and pepper. Shape the mixture into eight equal patties of two-inch.

Grease an iron skillet with oil.

Add the patties. Cook for six minutes on each side.

Nutrition:

Calories: 87.6 Protein: 11.3g Carbs: 0.2gFat: 7.5g Fiber: 0.1g

No-Bread Breakfast Sandwich

Preparation Time: Fifteen minutes

Cooking Time: Thirty minutes

Servings: Two servings

Ingredients

Two tbsps. of butter

Four large eggs

Pepper and salt

One ounce of deli ham (smoked)

Two ounces of cheddar cheese (cut in slices)

Few drops of Tabasco

Directions:

Heat the butter in an iron skillet. Add the eggs. Fry each side for two minutes. Add pepper and salt.

Take a fried egg. Add ham and cheese. Top with another fried egg.

Repeat for the other fried eggs.

Place the sandwich in the pan for one minute.

Sprinkle some Tabasco from the top.

Serve hot.

Nutrition:

Calories: 356.3

Protein: 20.3g

Carbs: 2.1g

Fat: 31.1g

Fiber: 0.2g

Baked Eggs

Preparation Time: Twenty minutes

Cooking Time: Thirty minutes

Servings: One serving

Ingredients

Three ounces of beef (ground)

Two large eggs

Two ounces of cheese (shredded)

Directions:

Preheat your oven at two hundred degrees Celsius.

Arrange the ground beef as the base in a baking dish.

Make two holes in the beef base. Crack the eggs in the holes.

Sprinkle cheese from the top.

Bake for fifteen minutes.

Let the baked eggs sit for five minutes.

Nutrition:

Calories: 497.6

Protein: 42.1g

Carbs: 2.1g

Fat: 34.5g

Fiber: 0.3g

Cured Salmon With Chives and Scrambled Eggs

Preparation Time: Fifteen minutes

Cooking Time: Thirty minutes

Servings: Two servings

Ingredients

Two large eggs

Two tbsps. of butter

One-fourth cup of whipping cream

One tbsp. of chives (chopped)

Two ounces of cured salmon

Pepper and salt

Directions:

Begin with whisking the eggs in a bowl.

Heat the butter in a pan. Add the eggs. Add the cream. Stir for three minutes.

Simmer for five minutes. Keep stirring for making the eggs creamy.

Add salt, chopped chives, and pepper.

Serve the eggs with cured salmon.

Nutrition:

Calories: 730.2

Protein: 49.6g

Carbs: 2.1g

Fat: 61.3g

Fiber: 0.1g

Eggs Benedict on Avocados

Preparation Time: Twenty minutes

Cooking Time: Thirty minutes

Servings: Four servings

Ingredients

For the hollandaise:

Three egg yolks

One tbsp. of lemon juice

Pepper and salt

Eight tbsps. of butter (unsalted)

For the eggs:

Two avocados (pitted, skinned)

Four large eggs

Five ounces of salmon (smoked)

Directions:

Add the butter in a bowl. Microwave for twenty seconds.

Add lemon juice and egg yolks. Use a hand blender for properly blending the mixture. Keep blending until a white layer forms. Add pepper and salt. Blend for two minutes.

Boil water in a saucepan. Crack the eggs in a small cup. Crack one egg at a time. Slide the eggs gently into the water. Cook for four minutes.

Cut the avocados in half. Add an egg on top of each avocado slice. Add hollandaise sauce from the top.

Add smoked salmon by the side.

Serve immediately.

Nutrition:

Calories: 523.6 Protein: 17.6g Carbs: 3.1gFat: 49.3g Fiber: 7.1g

CHAPTER 5:

Seafood / Fish

Keto Baked Salmon with Lemon and Butter

Preparation Time: 10 minutes

Cooking Time: 30 minutes

Servings: 3

Ingredients:

1-pound salmon

1 lemon

3 oz. butter

1 tablespoon olive oil

Ground black pepper and sea salt to taste

Directions:

Grease a large-sized baking dish with the olive oil and preheat your oven to 400°F.

Place the salmon on the baking dish, preferably skin-side down. Generously season with pepper and salt to taste.

Thinly slice the lemon and place the slices over the salmon. Cover the fish with ½ of the butter, preferably in very thin slices. Bake until the salmon flakes easily with a fork and is opaque, for 25 to 30 minutes, on middle rack.

Now, over moderate heat in a small sauce pan; heat the remaining butter until it begins to bubble. Immediately remove the pan from heat; set aside and let cool a bit. Gently add in some of the freshly squeezed lemon juice. Serve the cooked fish with some of the prepared lemon butter and enjoy.

Nutrition:

576 Calories 46g Total Fat 22g Saturated Fat 1.3g Total Carbohydrates 0.4g Dietary Fiber

0.4g Sugars 31g Protein

Ketogenic Spicy Oyster

Preparation Time: 10 minutes

Cooking Time: 5 minutes

Servings: 2

Ingredients:

12 oysters shucked

1 tablespoon olive oil

7-8 basil leaves, fresh

1 tablespoon garlic chili paste

1/8 teaspoon salt

Directions:

Combine olive oil with garlic chili paste and salt in a medium size mixing bowl; mix well.

Add oysters into the prepared sauce; turning them several times until thoroughly coated.

Create a bed for the oysters to cook by spreading the basil leaves out on an oven-safe dish.

Transfer the oysters and sauce over the bed of basil leaves; spreading them in a single layer on the dish.

Turn on the broiler over high-heat.

Place the dish on top rack (approximately a few inches away from the broiler) and broil for a few minutes.

Once done; immediately remove them from the oven. Serve hot and enjoy.

Nutrition:

102 Calories 8g Total Fat

2.5g Saturated Fat 2g Total Carbohydrates

0g Dietary Fiber 0.3g Sugars 4g Protein

Garlic Lime Mahi-Mahi

Preparation Time: 15 minutes

Cooking Time: 10 minutes + 30 minutes marination

Servings: 4

Ingredients:

4 Mahi-Mahi filets (approximately 1 to 1 ¼ pounds)

Zest and juice of 1 large lime, fresh

¼ cup avocado oil

3 cloves garlic, minced

1/8 teaspoon each of ground black pepper and fine grain sea salt

Directions:

For Marinade: Thoroughly combine the entire ingredients (except the filets) together in a small-sized mixing bowl. Pour the mixture on top of filets in a large zip-lock bag or large shallow dish. Let marinate for 30 minutes, at room temperature.

Pour the marinade into a large sauté pan (preferably with a cover) and heat it over medium heat. Once hot; carefully add the filets into the hot pan; cover and cook the filets for a couple of minutes, until cooked through.

Immediately remove the sauté pan from heat; set aside and let rest for 5 minutes, covered. Serve warm and enjoy.

Nutrition:

248 Calories

14g Total Fat

1.7g Saturated Fat

0.7g Total Carbohydrates

0.1g Dietary Fiber

0g Sugars

24g Protein

Fish and Leek Sauté

Preparation Time: 15 minutes

Cooking Time: 10 minutes

Servings: 2

Ingredients:

1 leek, chopped

2 trout fillets, diced (approximately 8 oz.)

1 tablespoon tamari soy sauce

1 teaspoon ginger, grated

1 tablespoon avocado oil

Salt to taste

Directions:

Over moderate heat in a large skillet; heat the avocado oil until hot. Once done; add and sauté the chopped leek for a few minutes, until turn soften.

Immediately add the diced trout with grated ginger, tamari sauce and salt to taste.

Continue to sauté the trout until it's not translucent anymore and cooked through.

Serve immediately and enjoy.

Nutrition:

175 Calories

7.6g Total Fat

1.5g Saturated Fat

5.2g Total Carbohydrates

0.8g Dietary Fiber

1.7g Sugars

21g Protein

Smoked Salmon Salad

Preparation Time: 5 minutes

Cooking Time: 0 minutes

Servings: 1

Ingredients:

2 oz. smoked salmon

1 lemon slice

4 olives

1 teaspoon pink peppercorns, crushed lightly

A handful of arugula salad leaves, fresh

Directions:

Place the olives and salad leaves into a large plate or shallow bowl.

Arrange the smoked salmon over the salad.

Sprinkle the top of smoked salmon with lightly crushed pink peppercorns.

Garnish your salad with a lemon slice; serve immediately and enjoy.

Nutrition:

149 Calories

5.2g Total Fat

1.4g Saturated Fat

4g Total Carbohydrates

1.7g Dietary Fiber

3.4g Sugars

11g Protein

Keto Baked Salmon with Pesto

Preparation Time: 10 minutes

Cooking Time: 30 minutes

Servings: 2

Ingredients:

1 oz. green pesto

½ pound salmon

Pepper and salt to taste

For Green sauce:

¼ cup Greek yogurt

1 oz. green pesto

¼ teaspoon garlic

Pepper and salt to taste

Directions:

Preheat your oven to 400°F.

Arrange the salmon in a well-greased baking dish, preferably skin-side down. Spread the pesto over the salmon and then, sprinkle with pepper and salt to taste.

Bake in the preheated oven until the salmon flakes easily with a fork, for 25 to 30 minutes.

In the meantime, stir the entire sauce ingredients together in a large bowl. Serve the cooked fish with some of the prepared sauce and enjoy.

Nutrition:

274 Calories 21g Total Fat

3.9g Saturated Fat 2.9g Total Carbohydrates

0.6g Dietary Fiber 1.7g Sugars 26g Protein

Roasted Salmon with Parmesan Dill Crust

Preparation Time: 10 minutes

Cooking Time: 10 minutes

Servings: 2

Ingredients:

½ pound salmon; cut into pieces

1 tablespoon dill weed

¼ cup cottage cheese

1 tablespoon olive oil

¼ cup parmesan cheese, grated

Directions:

Preheat your oven to 450°F.

Combine cottage cheese with parmesan cheese, olive oil and dill in a large-sized mixing bowl; mix well.

Line a large-sized baking sheet with aluminum foil and then, arrange the salmon pieces on it.

Smear ½ of the cottage cheese mix over the salmon.

Roast in the preheated oven until the fish flakes easily and crust is brown, for 10 minutes.

Serve the cooked fish with the remaining prepared sauce and enjoy.

Nutrition:

352 Calories

22g Total Fat

6.6g Saturated Fat

5.7g Total Carbohydrates

1.5g Dietary Fiber

0.5g Sugars

33g Protein

Keto Fried Salmon with Broccoli and Cheese

Preparation Time: 15 minutes

Cooking Time: 25 minutes

Servings: 3

Ingredients:

¾ pound salmon; cut into pieces

3 tablespoons butter

½ pound broccoli; cut into small florets

2 oz. cheddar cheese, grated

Pepper and salt to taste

1 lime

Directions:

Preheat your oven using the broiler settings, to 400°F.

Let the broccoli florets to simmer for a couple of minutes, preferably in lightly salted water. Ensure that the broccoli maintains its delicate color and chewy texture; drain well.

Now arrange the broccoli in a baking dish, preferably well-greased. Add butter and pepper to taste.

Sprinkle with cheese and bake in the preheated oven until the cheese turns golden in color, for 15 to 20 minutes.

Now, over moderate heat in a large saucepan; heat the butter until completely melted and fry the salmon pieces for a couple of minutes per side. Serve the pan-fried salmon with baked broccoli and enjoy.

Nutrition:

392 Calories 25g Total Fat

11.8g Saturated Fat 5.8g Total Carbohydrates

3.4g Dietary Fiber 1.4g Sugars 31g Protein

CHAPTER 6:

Beef, Lamb And Pork

Herbed Beef Tenderloin

Preparation time: 15 minutes

Cooking time: 30 minutes

Servings: 6

Ingredients

4 garlic cloves, minced - ½ cup fresh parsley, chopped

1/3 cup fresh oregano, chopped

2 tablespoons fresh thyme, chopped

2 tablespoons fresh rosemary, chopped

2 teaspoons fresh lemon zest, grated

6 tablespoons olive oil - 2 tablespoons fresh lemon juice

½ teaspoon red pepper flakes

Salt and ground black pepper, to taste

1¾ pounds grass-fed beef tenderloin, silver skin removed

Directions:

Add all ingredients except for beef tenderloin in a large bowl and mix well. Add the beef tenderloin and coat with the herb mixture generously. Refrigerate to marinate for about 30–45 minutes. Preheat the oven to 425°F. Remove the beef tenderloin from the bowl and arrange onto a baking sheet. Bake for approximately 30 minutes. Remove the beef tenderloin from oven and place onto a cutting board for about 15–20 minutes before slicing. With a sharp knife, cut the beef tenderloin into desired sized slices and serve.

Nutrition

Calories 415   Net Carbs 2.2 g   Fiber 2.4 g   Sugar 0.4 g   Protein 39.2 g

Steak with Cheese Sauce

Preparation time: 15 minutes

Cooking time: 17 minutes

Servings: 3

Ingredients

Steak

2 tablespoons fresh oregano, chopped

½ tablespoon garlic, minced

1 tablespoon fresh lemon peel, grated

½ teaspoon red pepper flakes, crushed

Salt and ground black pepper, to taste

1 (1-pound) (1-inch thick) grass-fed boneless beef top sirloin steak

Cheese Sauce

2 tablespoons unsalted butter

2 garlic cloves, minced

1 tablespoons almond flour

½ cup homemade beef broth

½ teaspoon dried basil

¼ teaspoon dried oregano

½ ounce cream cheese, softened

¼ cup Parmesan cheese, grated

¼ cup heavy cream

Salt and ground black pepper, to taste

Directions:

Preheat the gas grill to medium heat. Lightly, grease the grill grate.

In a bowl, add the oregano, garlic, lemon peel, red pepper flakes, salt, and black pepper, and mix well.

Rub the steak with garlic mixture evenly.

Place the steak onto the grill and cook, covered for about 12–17 minutes, flipping occasionally.

Remove the steak from the grill and place onto a cutting board for about 10 minutes.

For cheese sauce: Melt butter in the wok over medium heat and sauté the garlic for about 1 minute.

Stir in the flour and cook for about 1 minute, stirring continuously.

Stir in broth and dried herbs and cook for about 1 minute, stirring continuously.

Stir in cream cheese, Parmesan cheese and heavy cream and cook for about 1 minute, stirring continuously.

Stir in salt and black pepper and remove from the heat.

With a sharp knife, cut the steak into desired sized slices.

Divide steak slices onto serving plates and top with cheese sauce.

Serve immediately.

Nutrition

    Calories 461

    Net Carbs 2.7 g

    Total Fat 25.9 g

    Saturated Fat 12.8 g

    Cholesterol 180 mg

    Sodium 408 mg

    Total Carbs 4.5 g

    Fiber 1.8 g

    Sugar 0.5 g

    Protein 50.6 g

Steak with Pesto

Preparation time: 10 minutes

Cooking time: 10 minutes

Servings: 4

Ingredients

1 tablespoon butter

4 (6-ounce) grass-fed flank steaks

Salt and ground black pepper, to taste

½ cup pesto

Directions:

For steak: In a wok, melt the butter over medium-high heat and cook steaks with salt and black pepper for about 3–5 minutes per side.

Transfer the steaks onto serving plates and serve with the topping of pesto.

Nutrition

    Calories 490

    Net Carbs 1.5 g

    Total Fat 30 g

    Saturated Fat 10.2 g

    Cholesterol 109 mg

    Sodium 344 mg

    Total Carbs 2 g

    Fiber 0.5 g

    Sugar 2 g

    Protein 50.4 g

Herbed Lamb Chops

Preparation time: 10 minutes

Cooking time: 20 minutes

Servings: 4

Ingredients

1½ pounds grass-fed lamb loin chops, trimmed

1 tablespoon fresh lemon juice

¼ cup fresh parsley, chopped

2 tablespoons fresh mint leaves, chopped

1 tablespoon olive oil

Salt and ground black pepper, to taste

Directions:

Preheat grill to medium-high heat. Grease the grill grate.

In a bowl, add lamb loin chops, lemon juice, parsley, mint, oil, salt, and black pepper and mix well.

Place the chops onto the grill and cook for about 10 minutes per side or until desired doneness.

Serve hot.

Nutrition

- Calories 350
- Net Carbs 0.3 g
- Total Fat 16.1 g
- Saturated Fat 5 g
- Cholesterol 153 mg
- Sodium 172 mg
- Total Carbs 0.6 g
- Fiber 0.3 g
- Sugar 0.1 g   Protein 48 g

Stuffed Leg of Lamb

Preparation time: 20 minutes

Cooking time: 2 hours 5 minutes

Servings: 14

Ingredients

4 teaspoons olive oil, divided

¼ cup scallions, chopped

2 garlic cloves, chopped finely

1 cup fresh spinach leaves, shredded

2 tablespoons sun-dried tomatoes (in olive oil), drained and chopped finely

¼ cup fresh basil leaves, shredded

2 tablespoons pine nuts

2 teaspoons lemon pepper, divided

½ cup feta cheese, crumbled

1 (4-5-pound) grass-fed boneless leg of lamb, trimmed and butterflied

Directions:

Preheat the oven to 325°F. Arrange a greased rack into a roasting pan. In a medium wok, heat 2 teaspoons of the olive oil over medium heat and sauté the scallion and garlic for about 2 minutes. Stir in the spinach, sun-dried tomatoes, basil, pine nuts, and 1 teaspoon of the lemon pepper and cook for about 2–3 minutes, stirring frequently. Remove from the heat and stir in feta cheese. Set aside. Remove the strings from leg of lamb and open it. Place the stuffing in the center of meat evenly and roll to seal the filling.

Carefully, tie the leg of lamb with kitchen string. Coat the rolled leg of lamb with the remaining oil and sprinkle with 1 teaspoon of lemon pepper. Arrange the rolled leg of lamb into the prepared roasting pan. Roast for about 2 hours. Remove the leg of lamb from the oven and place onto a cutting board. With a piece of foil, cover the leg of lamb for 10 minutes before slicing. Cut into desired sized slices and serve.

Nutrition

Calories 340   Net Carbs 0.9 g   Fiber 0.3 g   Sugar 0.3 g   Protein 46.6 g

Grilled Pork Chops

Preparation time: 10 minutes

Cooking time: 12 minutes

Servings: 4

Ingredients

¼ cup fresh basil leaves, minced

2 garlic cloves, minced

2 tablespoons butter, melted

2 tablespoons fresh lemon juice

Salt and ground black pepper, as required

4 (6- to 8-ounce) bone-in pork loin chops

Directions:

In a baking dish, add the basil, garlic, butter, lemon juice, salt, and black pepper, and mix well.

Add the chops and generously coat with the mixture.

Cover the baking dish and refrigerate for about 30–45 minutes.

Preheat a gas grill to medium-high heat. Lightly, grease the grill grate.

Place chops onto the grill and cook for about 6 minutes per side or until desired doneness.

Serve hot.

Nutrition

    Calories 600

    Net Carbs 0.6 g

    Fiber 0.1 g

    Sugar 0.2 g

    Protein 38.5 g

Pork Chops in Cream Sauce

Preparation time: 15 minutes

Cooking time: 35 minutes

Servings: 4

Ingredients

2 tablespoons olive oil

4 large boneless rib pork chops

Salt, to taste

3 tablespoons yellow onion, chopped finely

2 tablespoons fresh rosemary, chopped

1/3 cup homemade chicken broth

1 tablespoon Dijon mustard

1 tablespoon unsalted butter

2/3 cup heavy cream

2 tablespoons sour cream

2 tablespoons fresh parsley, minced

Directions:

Heat the oil in a large wok over medium heat and sear the chops with the salt for about 3–4 minutes or until browned completely. With a slotted spoon, transfer the pork chops onto a plate and set aside. In the same wok, add the mushrooms, onion, and rosemary, and sauté for about 3 minutes.

Stir in the cooked chops, broth and bring to a boil.

Adjust the heat to low and cook, covered for about 20 minutes.

With a slotted spoon, transfer the pork chops onto a plate and set aside.

In the wok, add the butter, heavy cream, and sour cream, and stir until smooth. Stir in the cooked pork chops and cook for about 2–3 minutes or until heated completely. Serve hot.

Nutrition

Calories 727   Net Carbs 1.9 g   Fiber 1.1 g   Sugar 0.5 g   Protein 39.6 g

Sweet & Tangy Pork Tenderloin

Preparation time: 15 minutes

Cooking time: 22 minutes

Servings: 3

Ingredients

1 teaspoon fresh rosemary, minced

1 garlic clove, minced

1 tablespoon balsamic vinegar

1 tablespoon olive oil

1 teaspoon fresh lemon juice

1 teaspoon Dijon mustard

1 teaspoon Erythritol

Salt and ground black pepper, to taste

1 pound pork tenderloin

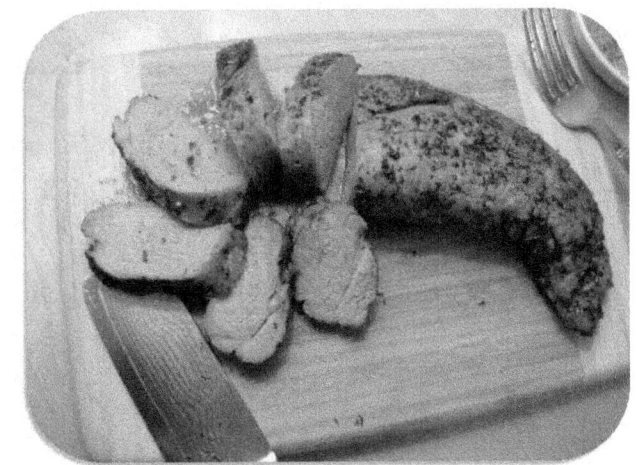

Directions:

Preheat oven to 400°F.

Grease a large rimmed baking sheet.

Add all ingredients except for pork tenderloin and cheese in a mixing bowl and beat until well combined.

Add the pork tenderloin and coat with the mixture generously.

Arrange the pork tenderloin onto the prepared baking sheet.

Bake for approximately 20–22 minutes.

Remove from the oven and place the pork tenderloin onto a cutting board for about 5 minutes.

With a sharp knife, cut the pork tenderloin into ¾-inch thick slices and serve with the topping of cheese.

Nutrition

Calories 262   Net Carbs 0.5 g   Fiber 0.3 g   Sugar 0.1 g   Protein 39.7 g

CHAPTER 7:

Poultry Recipes

Grilled Whole Chicken

Preparation time: 20 minutes

Cooking time: 20 minutes

Servings: 6

Ingredients

¼ cup butter, melted - 2 tablespoons fresh lemon juice

2 teaspoons fresh lemon zest, grated finely

1 teaspoon dried oregano, crushed

2 teaspoons paprika - 1 teaspoon onion powder

1 teaspoon garlic powder

Salt and ground black pepper, as required

1 (4-pound) grass-fed whole chicken, neck and giblets removed

Directions:

Preheat the grill to medium heat. Grease the grill grate. In a bowl, add the butter, lemon juice, lemon zest, oregano, spices, salt, and black pepper, and mix until well combined. Place chicken onto a large cutting board, breast-side down. With a sharp knife, cut along both sides of backbone and then remove the backbone. Now, flip the breast side of chicken up and open it like a book. With the palm of your hands, firmly press breast to flatten. Coat the whole chicken with the oil mixture generously. Arrange the chicken onto the grill and cook for about 16–20 minutes, flipping once halfway through. Remove from the grill and place the chicken onto a cutting board for about 5–10 minutes before carving. With a sharp knife, cut the chicken into desired-sized pieces and serve.

Nutrition

Calories 532   Net Carbs 0 g   Total Fat 17 g Fiber 0.5 g Sugar 0.5 g   Protein 88 g

Grilled Chicken Breast

Preparation time: 15 minutes

Cooking time: 14 minutes

Servings: 4

Ingredients

¼ cup balsamic vinegar

2 tablespoons olive oil

1½ teaspoons fresh lemon juice

½ teaspoon lemon-pepper seasoning

4 (6-ounce) grass-fed boneless skinless chicken breast halves, pounded slightly

Directions:

In a glass baking dish, place the vinegar, oil, lemon juice, and seasoning, and mix well.

Add the chicken breasts and coat with the mixture generously.

Refrigerate to marinate for about 25–30 minutes.

Preheat the grill to medium heat. Grease the grill grate.

Remove the chicken from bowl and discard the remaining marinade.

Place the chicken breasts onto the grill and cover with the lid.

Cook for about 5–7 minutes per side or until desired doneness.

Serve hot.

Nutrition

Calories 258

Net Carbs 0.3 g

Fiber 0.1 g

Sugar 0.1 g

Protein 36.1 g

Glazed Chicken Thighs

Ingredients

½ cup balsamic vinegar

1/3 cup low-sodium soy sauce

3 tablespoons Yacon syrup

4 tablespoons olive oil

3 tablespoons chili sauce

2 tablespoons garlic, minced

Salt and ground black pepper, as required

8 (6-ounce) grass-fed skinless chicken thighs

Preparation time: 15 minutes

Cooking time: 35 minutes

Servings: 8

Directions:

In a bowl, add all ingredients (except chicken thighs and sesame seeds) and beat until well combined.

In a large plastic zipper bag, add half of marinade and chicken thighs.

Seal the bag and shake to coat well.

Pace the bag in refrigerator for at least 1 hour, turning bag twice.

Reserve remaining marinade in the refrigerator until using.

Preheat your oven to 425°F. In a small pan, add reserved marinade over medium heat and bring to a boil. Cook for about 3–5 minutes, stirring occasionally. Remove the pan of sauce from heat and set aside to cool slightly.

Remove the chicken from the bag and discard excess marinade.

Arrange chicken thighs into a 9x13-inch baking dish in a single layer and coat with some of the cooked marinade. Bake for about 30 minutes, coating with the cooked marinade slightly after every 10 minutes. Serve hot.

Nutrition

Calories 406   Net Carbs 4.4 g   Total Fat 19.6 g Sugar 2.6 g   Protein 50 g

Bacon-Wrapped Chicken Breasts

Preparation time: 15 minutes

Cooking time: 33 minutes

Servings: 4

Ingredients

Chicken Marinade

3 tablespoons balsamic vinegar

3 tablespoons olive oil

2 tablespoons water

1 garlic clove, minced

1 teaspoon dried Italian seasoning

½ teaspoon dried rosemary

Salt and ground black pepper, as required

4 (6-ounce) grass-fed skinless, boneless chicken breasts

Stuffing

16 fresh basil leaves

1 large fresh tomato, sliced thinly

4 provolone cheese slices

8 bacon slices

¼ cup Parmesan cheese, grated freshly

Directions:

For marinade: In a bowl, add all ingredients (except chicken) and mix until well combined.

Place 1 chicken breast onto a smooth surface.

Hold a sharp knife parallel to work surface, slice the chicken breast horizontally, without cutting all the way through.

Repeat with the remaining chicken breasts.

Place the breasts in the bowl of marinade and toss to coat well.

Refrigerate, covered, for at least 30 minutes.

Preheat your oven to 500°F. Grease a baking dish.

Remove chicken breast from bowl and arrange onto a smooth surface.

Place 4 basil leaves onto the bottom half of a chicken breast. Followed by 2–3 tomato slices and 1 provolone cheese slice.

Now, fold the top half over filling.

Wrap the breast with 3 bacon slices and secure with toothpicks.

Repeat with the remaining chicken breasts and filling.

Arrange breasts into the prepared baking dish in a single layer.

Bake for about 30 minutes, flipping one halfway through.

Remove from the oven and sprinkle each chicken breast with Parmesan cheese evenly.

Bake for about 2–3 minutes more.

Serve hot.

Nutrition

Calories 633

Net Carbs 2.5 g

Total Fat 36 g

Fiber 0.3 g

Sugar 0.7 g

Protein 70.6 g

Chicken Parmigiana

Preparation time: 15 minutes

Cooking time: 26 minutes

Servings: 5

Ingredients

5 (6-ounce) grass-fed skinless, boneless chicken breasts

1 large organic egg, beaten

½ cup superfine blanched almond flour

¼ cup Parmesan cheese, grated

½ teaspoon dried parsley

½ teaspoon paprika

½ teaspoon garlic powder

Salt and ground black pepper, as required

¼ cup olive oil

1 cups sugar-free tomato sauce

5 ounces mozzarella cheese, thinly sliced

2 tablespoons fresh parsley, chopped

Directions:

Preheat your oven to 375°F.

Arrange 1 chicken breast between 2 pieces of parchment paper.

With a meat mallet, pound the chicken breast into ½-inch thickness

Repeat with the remaining chicken breasts.

Add the beaten egg into a shallow dish.

Place the almond flour, Parmesan, parsley, spices, salt, and black pepper in another shallow dish, and mix well.

Dip chicken breasts into the whipped egg and then coat with the flour mixture.

Heat the oil in a deep wok over medium-high heat and fry the chicken breasts for about 3 minutes per side.

With a slotted spoon, transfer the chicken breasts onto a paper towel-lined plate to drain.

In the bottom of a casserole dish, place about ½ cup of tomato sauce and spread evenly.

Arrange the chicken breasts over marinara sauce in a single layer.

Top with the remaining tomato sauce, followed by mozzarella cheese slices.

Bake for about 20 minutes or until done completely.

Remove from the oven and serve hot with the garnishing of parsley.

Nutrition

Calories 458

Net Carbs 5.4 g

Fiber 2.5 g

Sugar 3.7 g

Protein 50.4 g

Roasted Turkey

Preparation time: 15 minutes

Cooking time: 3 hours 30 minutes

Servings: 12

Ingredients

Marinade

1 (2-inch) piece fresh ginger, grated finely

3 large garlic cloves, crushed

1 green chili, chopped finely

1 teaspoon fresh lemon zest, grated finely

5 ounces plain Greek yogurt

3 tablespoons homemade tomato puree

2 tablespoons fresh lemon juice

1½ tablespoons garam masala

1 tablespoon ground cumin

2 teaspoons ground turmeric

Turkey

1 (9-pound) whole turkey, giblets and neck removed

Salt and ground black pepper, as required

1 garlic clove, halved

1 lime, halved

1 lemon, halved

Directions:

For marinade: In a bowl, mix together all ingredients.

With a fork, pierce the turkey completely.

In a large baking dish, place the turkey and rub with the marinade mixture evenly.

Refrigerate to marinate overnight.

Remove the turkey from refrigerator and set aside for about 30 minutes before cooking.

Preheat your oven to 390°F.

Sprinkle turkey with salt and black pepper evenly and stuff the cavity with garlic, lime, and lemon.

Arrange the turkey in a large roasting pan and roast for about 30 minutes.

Now, reduce the temperature of oven to 350°F.

Roast for about 3 hours. (If skin becomes brown during roasting, then cover with a piece of foil.)

Remove from the oven and palace the turkey onto a platter for about 15–20 minutes before carving.

With a sharp knife, cut the turkey into desired sized pieces and serve.

Nutrition

Calories 595

Net Carbs 2 g

Fiber 0.3 g

Sugar 1.2 g

Protein 100.3 g

Roasted Turkey Breast

Preparation time: 15 minutes

Cooking time: 2½ hours

Total time: 2¾ hours

Servings: 14

Ingredients

1 teaspoon onion powder

½ teaspoon garlic powder

Salt and ground black pepper, as required

1 (7-pound) bone-in turkey breast

1½ cups Italian dressing

Directions:

Preheat your oven to 325°F.

Grease a 13x9-inch baking dish.

In a bowl, add the onion powder, garlic powder, salt, and black pepper, and mix well.

Rub the turkey breast with the seasoning mixture generously.

Arrange the turkey breast into the prepared baking dish and top with the Italian dressing evenly.

Bake for about 2–2½ hours, coating with pan juices occasionally.

Remove from the oven and palace the turkey breast onto a platter for about 10–15 minutes before slicing.

With a sharp knife, cut the turkey breast into desired-sized slices and serve.

Nutrition

Calories 459 Net Carbs 2.8 g

Total Fat 23.3 g Fiber 0 g

Sugar 2.2 g   Protein 48.7 g

CHAPTER 8:

Salad Recipes

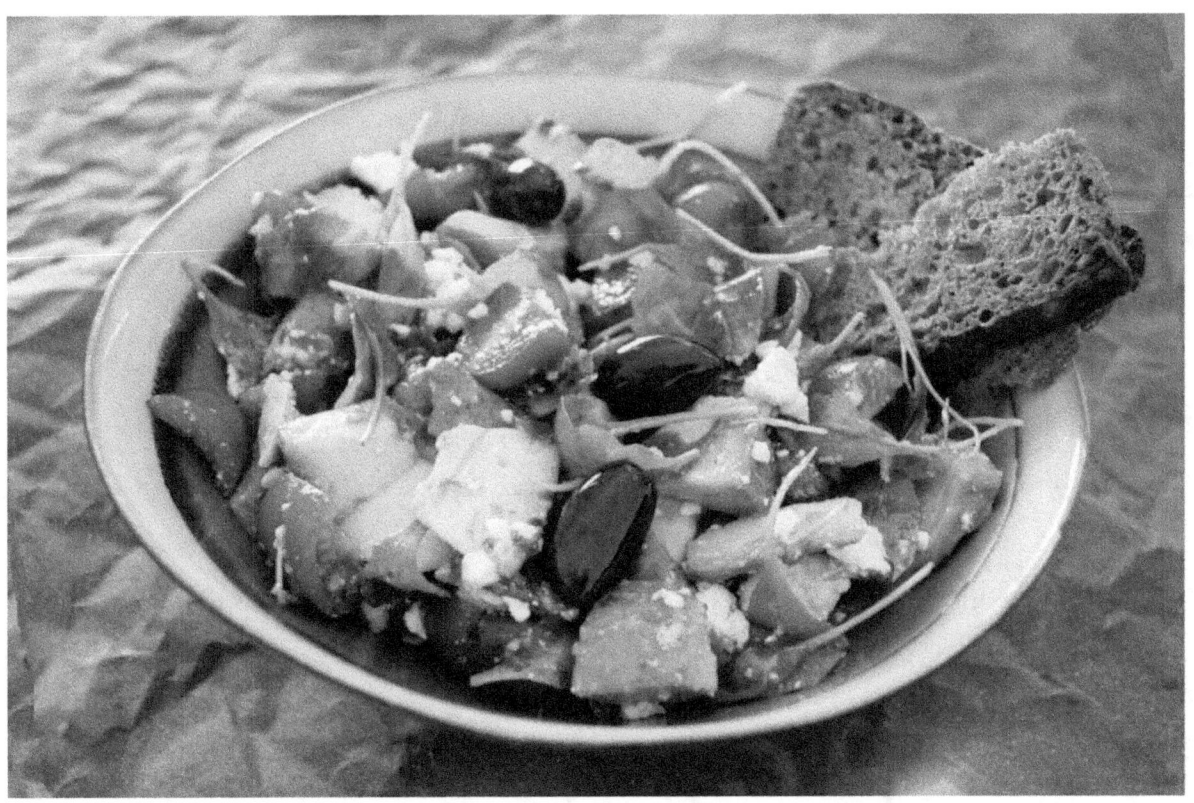

Roasted Brussels Sprouts Salad with Parmesan

Preparation Time: 10 minutes

Cooking Time: 15 minutes

Serving: 2

Ingredients:

1-pound Brussels sprouts

1 tablespoon olive oil

Pink Himalayan salt

Freshly ground black pepper

¼ cup shaved or grated Parmesan cheese

¼ cup whole, skinless hazelnuts

Directions:

Preheat the oven to 350°F. Line a baking sheet with a silicone baking mat or parchment paper.

Trim the bottom and core from each Brussels sprout with a small knife. This will release the leaves.

Put the leaves in a medium bowl; you can use your hands to release all the leaves fully.

Toss the leaves with the olive oil and season with pink Himalayan salt and pepper.

Spread the leaves in a single layer on the baking sheet—roast for 10 to 15 minutes, or until lightly browned and crisp.

Divide the roasted Brussels sprouts leaves between two bowls, top each with the shaved Parmesan cheese and hazelnuts, and serve.

If you don't have hazelnuts, use chopped almonds.

Nutrition:

Calories: 287

Fat: 19g

Carbs: 23g

Fiber: 10g

Protein: 14g

Wedge Salad

Preparation Time: 10 minutes

Cooking Time: 10 minutes

Serving: 2

Ingredients:

4 bacon slices

½ head iceberg lettuce halved

2 tablespoons blue cheese salad dressing (I use Trader Joe's Chunky Blue Cheese Dressing)

¼ cup blue cheese crumbles

½ cup halved grape tomatoes

Directions:

In a large skillet over medium-high heat, cook the bacon on both sides until crispy, about 8 minutes. Transfer the bacon to a paper towel-lined plate to drain and cool for 5 minutes. Transfer to a cutting board and chop the bacon.

Place the lettuce wedges on two plates. Top each with half of the blue cheese dressing, the blue cheese crumbles, the halved grape tomatoes, and the chopped bacon, and serve.

If you have a grill, you can drizzle each of your iceberg lettuce wedges with one tablespoon of olive oil, season with pink Himalayan salt and pepper, and grill each side for about 1 minute to add some smoky flavor. Then dress the lettuce wedges as instructed.

Nutrition:

Calories: 278

Fat: 20g

Carbs: 9g

Fiber: 3g

Protein: 15g

Mexican Egg Salad

Preparation Time: 15 minutes

Cooking Time: 10 minutes

Serving: 2

Ingredients:

4 large eggs

½ cup shredded cheese (I use Mexican blend), divided

1 jalapeño

1 avocado halved

Pink Himalayan salt

Freshly ground black pepper

2 tablespoons chopped fresh cilantro

Directions:

Preheat the oven to 350°F. Line a baking sheet with parchment paper or a silicone baking mat.

To Make The Hardboiled Eggs

In a medium saucepan, cover the eggs with water. Place over high heat, and bring the water to a boil. Once it is boiling, turn off the heat, cover, and leave on the burner for 10 to 12 minutes. Use a slotted spoon to remove the eggs from the pan and run them under cold water for 1 minute or submerge in an ice bath. Gently tap the shells and peel. (I like to run cold water over my hands as I peel the shells off.)

To Make The Cheese Chips

While the eggs are cooking, put 2 (¼-cup) mounds of shredded cheese on the prepared pan and bake for about 7 minutes, or until the edges are brown and the middle has fully melted. Remove the cheese chips from the oven and allow to cool for 5 minutes; they will be floppy when they first come out but will crisp as they cool. In a medium bowl, chop the hardboiled eggs. Stem, rib, seed, and dice the jalapeño and add it to the eggs. Mash the avocado with a fork—season with pink Himalayan salt and pepper. Add the avocado and cilantro to the eggs and stir to combine. Place the cheese chips on two plates, top with the egg salad, and serve.

Nutrition:

Calories: 359 Fat: 29g Carbs: 8g Fiber: 5g Protein: 21g

Blue Cheese and Bacon Kale Salad

Preparation Time: 10 minutes

Cooking Time: 10 minutes

Serving: 2

Ingredients:

4 bacon slices

2 cups stemmed and chopped fresh kale

1 tablespoon vinaigrette salad dressing (I use Primal Kitchen Greek Vinaigrette)

Pinch pink Himalayan salt

Pinch freshly ground black pepper

¼ cup pecans

¼ cup blue cheese crumbles

Directions:

In a medium skillet over medium-high heat, cook the bacon on both sides until crispy, about 8 minutes. Transfer the bacon to a paper towel-lined plate.

Meanwhile, in a large bowl, massage the kale with the vinaigrette for 2 minutes. Add the pink Himalayan salt and pepper. Let the kale sit while the bacon cooks, and it will get even softer.

Chop the bacon and pecans, and add them to the bowl. Sprinkle in the blue cheese.

Toss well to combine, portion onto two plates, and serve.

Chopped almonds can replace the chopped pecans.

Nutrition:

Calories: 353

Fat: 29g

Carbs: 10g

Fiber: 3g

Protein: 16g

Chopped Greek Salad

Preparation Time: 10 minutes

Cooking Time: 10 minutes

Serving: 2

Ingredients:

2 cups chopped romaine

½ cup halved grape tomatoes

¼ cup sliced black olives (like Kalamata)

¼ cup feta cheese crumbles

2 tablespoons vinaigrette salad dressing (I use Primal Kitchen Greek Vinaigrette)

Pink Himalayan salt

Freshly ground black pepper

1 tablespoon olive oil

Directions:

In a large bowl, combine the romaine, tomatoes, olives, feta cheese, and vinaigrette.

Season with pink Himalayan salt and pepper, drizzle with the olive oil and toss to combine.

Divide the salad between two bowls and serve.

VARIATIONS

With Greek salad, there are so many great flavors you can add:

Red onion or finely chopped cucumbers for additional crunch and freshness, and chopped pepperoncini for a zesty kick.

Finely chopped Genoa salami and pepperoni are good choices.

You could replace the feta cheese with goat cheese.

Nutrition:

Calories: 202 Fat: 19g

Carbs: 4g Fiber: 2g Protein: 4g

Mediterranean Cucumber Salad

Preparation Time: 10 minutes

Cooking Time: 15 minutes

Serving: 2

Ingredients:

1 large cucumber, peeled and finely chopped

½ cup halved grape tomatoes

¼ cup halved black olives (I used Kalamata)

¼ cup crumbled feta cheese

Pink Himalayan salt

Directions:

Freshly ground black pepper

Two tablespoons vinaigrette salad dressing (I use Primal Kitchen Greek Vinaigrette)

In a large bowl, combine the cucumber, tomatoes, olives, and feta cheese—season with pink Himalayan salt and pepper. Add the dressing and toss to combine.

Divide the salad between two bowls and serve.

This salad can be eaten immediately, of course, but I think it is even better if you cover it with wrap and put it in the fridge to let the dressing marinate the salad ingredients for a few hours.

Nutrition:

Per Serving

Calories: 152

Fat: 13g

Carbs: 6g

Fiber: 2g

Protein: 4g

Avocado Egg Salad Lettuce Cups

Preparation Time: 15 minutes

Cooking Time: 15 minutes

Serving: 2

Ingredients:

4 large eggs - 1 avocado halved - Pink Himalayan salt

Freshly ground black pepper - ½ teaspoon freshly squeezed lemon juice

4 butter lettuce cups washed and patted dry with paper towels or a clean dish towel

2 radishes, thinly sliced

Directions:

TO MAKE THE HARDBOILED EGGS

1. In a medium saucepan, cover the eggs with water. Place over high heat, and bring the water to a boil. Once it is boiling, turn off the heat, cover, and leave on the burner for 10 to 12 minutes.

2. Remove the eggs with a slotted spoon and run them under cold water for 1 minute or submerge them in an ice bath.

3. Then gently tap the shells and peel. Run cold water over your hands as you remove the shells.

TO MAKE THE EGG SALAD

1. In a medium bowl, chop the hardboiled eggs.

2. Add the avocado to the bowl, and mash the flesh with a fork. Season with pink Himalayan salt and pepper, add the lemon juice and stir to combine.

3. Place the four lettuce cups on two plates. Top the lettuce cups with the egg salad and the slices of radish and serve.

VARIATIONS

For this recipe, you can incorporate additional ingredients that you may have in your refrigerator or pantry: Add a guacamole vibe to your egg salad with chopped jalapeño and red onion.

Chopped bacon adds appealing texture to your egg salad, or add slices of crisp bacon to your lettuce cups. You could also use romaine hearts or baby cos lettuce.

Nutrition:

Calories: 258 Fat: 20g Carbs: 8g Fiber: 5g Protein: 15g

CHAPTER 9:

Vegetables

Avocado Chips

Preparation Time: 4 minutes

Cooking Time: 8 minutes

Servings: 2

Ingredients:

De-seeded, peeled, sliced avocado: 1

Panko breadcrumbs: ½ cup

All-purpose flour: ¼ cup

Large beaten egg: 1

Water: 1 tsp.

Kosher salt: ¼ tsp.

Ground Black pepper: ½ tsp.

Cooking spray.

Directions:

First, preheat the air fryer to 400 degrees F. spray basket with cooking spray

Combine flour and salt in a container, egg and water in another, and panko breadcrumbs in the last container. Dredge avocado slices in each, respectively.

Air fry for 4 minutes, flip the sides and again fry until golden brown.

Nutrition:

Energy: 320 g, Carbs: 40 g, Proteins: 9.2 g Fats: 18 g Sodium: 464 mg

Parmesan Zucchini Fries

Preparation Time: 5 minutes

Cooking Time: 20 minutes

Servings: 2

Ingredients:

Thinly sliced Zucchini: 1

Large beaten egg: 1

Grated Parmesan cheese: ¾ cup

Panko breadcrumbs: 1 cup

Directions:

First, preheat the air fryer at 350 degrees F.

Mix panko breadcrumbs and parmesan cheese. Dip zucchini in egg and then coat with panko breadcrumbs mixture. Gently press to firm the coating.

Air fry the zucchini fries for 10 minutes, shake the air fryer basket, and again air fry for 5 minutes.

Serve with coleslaw. Relish.

Nutrition:

Energy: 160 calories

Carbs: 21 g

Proteins: 10.9 g

Fats: 6.5 g

Sodium: 385 mg

Tofu with Peanut Dipping Sauce

Preparation Time: 5 minutes

Cooking Time: 17 minutes

Servings: 16

Ingredients:

Cubed Tofu: 16 oz.

All-purpose flour: 1 and ½ cup

Kosher salt: ½ tsp.

Freshly ground black pepper: ½ tsp.

Olive oil spray

For dipping sauce

Low sodium peanut butter: ¼ cup

Minced garlic: 1 tsp.

Light soy sauce: 12 tbsp.

Fresh lime juice: 1 tbsp.

Brown sugar: 1 tsp.

Water: 1/3 cup

Chopped roasted peanuts: 2 tbsp.

Directions:

Combine all-purpose flour with salt and pepper. Toss the tofu cubes with flour mixture and spray with oil.

Preheat the air fryer at 390 degrees F.

Transfer the tofu to the air fryer basket. Air fry for about 10 to 12 minutes or until golden brown.

Meanwhile, prepare dipping sauce by mixing all the dipping sauce ingredients and refrigerate.

Serve tofu with peanut dipping sauce. Relish.

Nutrition:

Energy: 255 calories Carbs: 21.1 g Protein: 12.5 g Fats: 14 g Sodium: 455 mg

Cream Cheese Mini Multi Sweet Peppers

Preparation Time: 7 minutes

Cooking Time: 15 minutes

Servings: 4 to 6

Ingredients:

Bulk Italian sausage: 8 ounces

Petite Multi-colored sweet pepper: 1 package

Softened cream cheese: 1 package

Divided olive oil: 2 tbsp.

Shredded Cheddar cheese: ½ cup

Crumbled blue cheese: 1 tbsp.

Finely chopped fresh chives: 1 tbsp.

Minced garlic cloves: 1 clove

Powdered black pepper: ¼ tsp.

Panko breadcrumbs: 2 tbsp.

Directions:

Bring to simmer the sausage in a skillet until crumbled.

Preheat the air fryer to 350 degrees F.

Split the multi-colored sweet pepper lengthwise into 2 halves. Paint with olive oil slightly and air fry for 3 to 5 minutes.

Meanwhile, whisk together sausage, cream cheese, cheddar cheese, blue cheese, chives, garlic, and black pepper. Now, in another bowl, mix panko breadcrumbs with olive oil.

Scoop in the cheese mixture into the split sweet peppers and dredge with panko breadcrumbs.

Air fry for 5 minutes again, shake and again fry for 3 minutes. Serve with favorite dipping. Relish.

Nutrition:

Energy: 100 calories

Carbs: 2.5 g Proteins: 3.6 g Fats: 8.6 g Sodium: 160 mg

Corn On the Cob

Preparation Time: 4 minutes

Cooking Time: 15 minutes

Servings: 2

Ingredients:

Sliced Corn ears: 2

Mayonnaise: ¼ cup

Crumbled cojita cheese: 2 tsp.

Lemon juice: 1 tsp.

Chili powder: ¼ tsp.

Fresh Cilantro: 4 sprigs

Directions:

First, preheat the air fryer to 400 degrees F for 3 mins.

Whisk together mayonnaise, lime juice, chili powder, and cojita cheese. Dip each corn in the mixture.

Now, air fry in the preheated air fryer for 8 minutes. Flip the sides and again fry for 5 minutes.

Nutrition:

Energy: 145 calories

Carbs: 9.4 g

Proteins: 2 g

Fats: 12 g

Sodium: 103 mg

Corn Nuts

Preparation Time: 3 minutes

Cooking Time: 20 minutes

Servings: 2

Ingredients:

Goya giant white corn: 14 ounce

Vegetable oil: 3 tbsp.

Kosher salt: 1 ½ tsp.

Directions:

Dwell the corn in water for overnight.

Drain & pat dry with a paper towel.

Preheat the air fryer to 400 F.

Coat the corn with oil and salt, transfer to air fryer basket, and air fry for 10 minutes. Jerk the basket and fry for 7 minutes more. Relish

Nutrition:

Energy: 225 calories,

Carbs: 35.9 g,

Proteins: 6 g,

Fats: 7.5 g

Sodium: 438 mg

Toasted Broccoli and Cauliflower

Preparation Time: 4 minutes

Cooking Time: 22 minutes

Servings: 6

Ingredients:

Sliced Cauliflower: 3 cups

Diced Broccoli: 3 cups

Garlic powder: ½ tsp.

Sea salt: ¼ tsp.

Paprika: ¼ tsp.

Ground black pepper: 1/8 tsp.

Olive oil: 2 tbsp.

Directions:

First, preheat the air fryer at 400 degrees F.

Combine broccoli, cauliflower, olive oil, paprika, sea salt, black pepper, and garlic powder.

Pour the mixture in the preheated air fryer basket and air fry for 12 minutes. Jerk and again fry for 6 minutes.

Nutrition:

Energy: 69 calories

Carbs: 5.8 g

Proteins: 2.4 g

Fats: 4.7 g

Sodium: 104 mg

Air Fried, Roasted Okra

Preparation Time: 3 minutes

Cooking Time: 6 minutes

Servings: 4

Ingredients:

Sliced okra: ½ pound

Olive oil: 1 tsp.

Salt and black pepper: to taste

Directions:

Preheat the air fryer at 350 degrees F for 5 min.

Season okra with olive oil, pepper, and salt.

Air fry for mins, toss and again air fry for 3 mins. Relish.

Nutrition:

Energy: 112 calories,

Carbs: 16 g,

Proteins: 4.7 g,

Fats: 5 g,

Sodium 600 mg

Vegetable Pakoras

Preparation Time: 15 minutes

Cooking Time: minutes 30

Servings: 8

Ingredients:

Diced cauliflower: 2 cups

Minced yellow potatoes: 1 cup

Chickpea flour: 1 ¼ cups

Chopped red onion: ½

Minced garlic clove: 1

Curry powder: 1 tsp.

Coriander: 1 tsp.

Cumin: ½ tsp.

Powdered cayenne pepper: ½ tsp.

Water: ¾ cup

Directions:

Combine cauliflower, red onion, potatoes, garlic, chickpea flour, salt, coriander, cayenne, cumin, and water in a container and let it rest for 10 to 12 mins.

Preheat the air fryer to 350 degrees F for 3 mins.

Spray the air fryer basket with cooking spray. Place cauliflower mixture into basket via a scoop.

Air fry for 8 mins, turn the sides and again cook for 5 mins. Serve with sauce. Relish.

Nutrition:

Energy: 80 calories

Carbs: 14.4 g

Proteins: 4.3 g

Fats: 1.1 g

Sodium: 890 mg

Cauliflower Rice

Preparation Time: 20 minutes

Cooking Time: 8 minutes

Servings: 2

Ingredients:

1 head of cauliflower

1 tbsp. Of olive oil or grass-fed butter

Salt to taste

Directions:

Slice the cauliflower into small pieces with a sharp knife, add in a food processor, and process it until fully broken.

If any pieces are left unprocessed, put them back in and process again.

Preheat a large pan and heat olive oil in it.

Add in your processed cauliflower with a pinch of salt.

Cover and cook for 4-8 minutes.

Then, serve warm.

Nutrition:

Calories: 204 kcal

Total Fat: 11g

Total Carbs: 4.2g

Protein: 1.5g

Keto Mushroom Soup

Preparation Time: 1 ½ hour

Cooking Time: 15 minutes

Servings: 4

Ingredients:

31 ounces of chicken broth

11 mushrooms

2 crushed garlic cloves

2 cups of heavy whipping cream

1 tablespoon of sherry

1 diced onion

1 teaspoon of salt

1 teaspoon of black pepper

½ cup of butter

½ teaspoon of thyme

¼ cup of vegetable stock

Directions:

Slice 9 mushrooms, and slice 2 separately.

In a heated pan, add in the butter, then onions, garlic, and the sliced mushrooms. Sauté for 3-5 minutes.

Pour in chicken broth and vegetable stock and stir on high flame. Then, add in sherry, thyme, salt, and pepper.

Reduce your heat to a low level, and simmer for 5 more minutes.

Pour in the cream gently, and stir to thicken. Throw in your 2 sliced mushrooms and steam for a minute or two. You can serve this soup with Keto bread.

Nutrition:

Calories: 464 kcal Total Fat: 65.5g Total Carbs: 1.5g Protein: 13.5g

Broccoli Salmon

Preparation Time: 30 minutes

Cooking Time: 40 minutes

Servings: 3

Ingredients:

8 ounces of cooked salmon

2 celery stalks

1 tablespoon of olive oil

1 head of medium-sized broccoli

1 tablespoon of Brain octane

½ teaspoon of thyme

¼ teaspoon of curry powder

½ teaspoon of black pepper

½ teaspoon of salt

½ trimmed leak

¼ of an avocado

½ of an onion sliced

Directions:

Mix curry, thyme, pepper, salt, and set aside.

Slice avocado into small pieces.

Add in leek, broccoli, and celery in a saucepan and boil it until soft.

Drain excess water, leaving only about 1 cup of liquid. Using some saved water, blend the veggies in a blender halfway between smooth. Do not use up all the water. Then, put in the blended spices, and mix well.In a saucepan, pour oil, and sauté onion until soft, then add blended veggies. Then, add sliced avocado and let it steam. Add in salmon, steam for 1 minute, then serve hot with rice or alone.

Nutrition:

Calories: 374 kcal Total Fat: 20.5g Total Carbs: 14g Protein: 26.6g

CHAPTER 10:

Soup Recipes

Creamy Broccoli and Leek Soup

Preparation time: 5 minutes

Cooking time: 25 minutes

Servings: 4

Ingredients:

Ten ozs. broccoli

One leek

Eight ozs. cream cheese

Three ozs. butter

3 cups of water

One garlic clove

½ cup fresh basil

salt and pepper

Directions:

Rinse the leek and chop both parts finely. Slice the broccoli thinly.

Place the veggies in a pot and cover with water and then season them. Boil the water until the broccoli softens.

Add the florets and garlic, while lowering the heat.

Add in the cheese, butter, pepper, and basil. Blend until desired consistency: if too thick use water; if you want to make it thicker, use a little bit of heavy cream.

Nutrition:

Calories: 451 kcal Fats: 37 g Protein: 10 g Carbs: 4 g

Chicken Soup

Preparation time: 25 minutes

Cooking time: 80 mins

Servings: 4

Ingredients:

6 cups of water

One chicken

One medium carrot

One yellow onion

One bay leaf

One leek

Two garlic cloves

1 tbsp. dried thyme

½ cup white wine, dry (no, not for drinking)

1 tsp. peppercorns

salt and pepper

Directions:

Peel and cut your veggies. Brown them in oil in a big pot.

Split your chicken in half, down in the middle. Pour water and spices in the pot. Let it simmer for one hour.

Take out the chicken, save the meat, and toss away the bones.

Put the meat back in the pot, and let it simmer on medium heat for 20-25 mins again, while seasoning to your liking.

Nutrition:

Calories: 145 kcal Fats: 12 g Carbs: 1 g Protein: 8 g

Greek Egg and Lemon Soup with Chicken

Preparation time: 5 minutes

Cooking time: 30 minutes

Servings: 4

Ingredients:

4 cups of water

¾ lbs. cauli

1 lb. boneless chicken thighs

1/3 lb. butter

Four eggs

One lemon

2 tbsps. fresh parsley

One bay leaf

Two chicken bouillon cubes

salt and pepper

Directions:

Slice your chicken thinly and then place it in a saucepan while adding cold water and the cubes and bay leaf. Let the meat simmer for 10 mins before removing it and the bay leaf.

Grate your cauli and place it in a saucepan. Add butter and boil for a few minutes.

Beat your eggs and lemon juice in a bowl, while seasoning it.

Reduce the heat a bit and add the eggs, stirring continuously. Let simmer but don't boil.

Return the chicken.

Nutrition:

Calories: 582 kcal

Carbs: 4 g

Fats: 49 g

Protein: 31 g

Wild Mushroom Soup

Preparation Time: 10 mins

Cooking Time: 30 mins

Servings: 4

Ingredients:

Six ozs. the mix of portabella mushrooms, oyster mushrooms, and shiitake mushrooms

3 cups of water

One garlic clove

One shallot

Four ozs. butter

One chicken bouillon cube

½ lb. celery root

1 tbsp. white wine vinegar

1 cup heavy whipping cream

fresh parsley

Directions:

Clean, trim, and chop your mushrooms and celery. Do the same to your shallot and garlic.

Sauté your chopped veggies in butter over medium heat in a saucepan.

Add thyme, vinegar, chicken bouillon cube, and water as you bring to boil. Then let it simmer for 10-15 mins.

Add cream to them with an immersion blender until your desired consistency. Serve with parsley on top.

Nutrition:

Calories: 481 kcal

Fats: 47 g

Protein: 7 g

Carbs: 9 g

Roasted Butternut Squash Soup

This one is a little bit longer soup, based on its cooking time, but it's worth it, trust us. When you roast it and inhale the caramelized smell, you will know that you made the right choice.

Preparation Time: 15 minutes

Cooking Time: 30 minutes

Servings: 4

Ingredients:

One large butternut squash, cubed and peeled

One stalk celery, sliced

Two potatoes, peeled, chopped

One onion, chopped

One large carrot, chopped

3 tbsps. olive oil

1 tbsp. fresh thyme

25 ozs. chicken broth

1 tbsp. butter

salt and pepper

Directions:

Preheat your oven to 400°F. On a baking sheet, toss squash and potatoes with 2 tbsp. Oil and season to your taster. Roast for 20-25 mins.

In the meantime, melt your butter and the rest of the oil in a large pot over medium heat. Add the onion, celery, carrot, and cook for 5-8 mins. Season them, too.

Add roasted squash and potatoes. Then pour over the chicken broth. Simmer it for 10 mins using an immersion blender until the soup is creamy.

Garnish it with thyme.

Nutrition:

Calories: 254 kcal Fats: 15 g Carbs: 19 g Protein: 6 g

Zucchini Cream Soup

Preparation Time: 5 minutes

Cooking Time: 20 minutes

Servings: 4

Ingredients:

Three zucchinis

32 ozs. chicken broth

Two cloves garlic

2 tbsps. sour cream

½ small onion

parmesan cheese (for topping if desired)

Directions:

Combine your broth, garlic, zucchini, and onion in a large pot over medium heat until boiling.

Lower the heat, cover, and let simmer for 15-20 mins

Remove from heat and purée with an immersion blender while adding the sour cream and pureeing until smooth.

Season to taste and top with your cheese.

Nutrition:

Calories: 117 kcal

Fats: 9 g

Carbs: 3 g

Protein: 4 g

Cauli Soup

Preparation Time: 5 minutes

Cooking Time: 25 minutes

Servings: 6

Ingredients:

32 ozs. vegetable broth

One head cauli, diced

Two garlic cloves, minced

One onion, diced

½ tbsp. olive oil

salt and pepper

grated parmesan, sliced green onion for topping

Directions:

In a pot, heat oil over medium heat, while adding the onion and garlic. Then cook them for 4-5 mins.

Add in the cauli and vegetable broth. Boil it and then cover for 15-20 mins while covered.

Pour all contents of the pot into a blender and season it.

Blend until smooth. Top it with your cheese and green onion.

Nutrition:

Calories: 37 kcal

Fats: 1 g

Carbs: 3 g

Protein: 3 g

Thai Coconut Soup

Preparation Time: 10 Minutes

Cooking Time: 35 Minutes

Servings: 4

Ingredients:

Three chicken breasts

Nine ozs. coconut milk

Nine ozs. chicken broth

2/3 tbsps. chili sauce

18 ozs. water

2/3 tbsps. coconut aminos

2/3 ozs. lime juice

2/3 tsp. ground ginger

¼ cup red boat fish sauce

salt and pepper

Directions:

Slice up the chicken breasts thinly. Make them bite-sized.

In a large stockpot, mix your coconut milk, water, fish sauce, chili sauce, lime juice, ginger, coconut aminos, and broth. Bring to a boil.

Stir in chicken pieces. Then reduce the heat and cover pot, while simmering it for 30 mins.

Remove the basil leaves and season it.

Nutrition:

Calories: 227 kcal

Fats: 17 g

Carbs: 3 g

Protein: 19 g

Chicken Ramen Soup

Preparation Time: 10 Minutes

Cooking Time: 20 Minutes

Servings: 2

Ingredients:

One chicken breast

Two eggs

One zucchini, made into noodles

4 cups chicken broth

Two cloves of garlic, peeled and minced

2 tbsps. coconut aminos

3 tbsps. avocado oil

1 tbsp. ginger

Directions:

Pan-fry the chicken in avocado oil in a pan until brown.

Hard boil your eggs and slice them in half.

Add chicken broth to a large pot and simmer with the garlic, coconut aminos, and ginger. Then add in the zucchini noodles for 4-5 mins.

Put the broth into a bowl, top it with eggs and chicken slices, and season to your liking.

Nutrition:

Calories: 478 kcal

Fats: 39 g

Carbs: 3 g

Protein: 31 g

Egg Drop Soup

Preparation Time: 5 Minutes

Cooking Time: 15 Minutes

Servings: 2

Ingredients:

3 cups chicken broth

2 cups Swiss chard chopped

Two eggs whisked

1 tsp. grated ginger

1 tsp. ground oregano

2 tbsps. coconut aminos

salt and pepper

Directions:

Heat your broth in a saucepan.

Slowly drizzle in the eggs while stirring slowly.

Add the Swiss chard, grated ginger, oregano, and coconut aminos. Next, season it and let it cook for 5-10 mins.

Nutrition:

Calories: 225 kcal

Fats: 19 g

Carbs: 4 g

Protein: 11 g

CHAPTER 11:

Dessert

Sugar-Free Lemon Bars

Preparation Time: 15 minutes

Cooking time: 45 minutes

Servings: 8

Ingredients:

½ cup butter, melted

1¾ cup almond flour, divided

1 cup powdered erythritol, divided

3 medium-size lemons

3 large eggs

Directions:

Prepare the parchment paper and baking tray. Combine butter, 1 cup of almond flour, ¼ cup of erythritol, and salt. Stir well. Place the mix on the baking sheet, press a little and put it into the oven (preheated to 350°F). Cook for about 20 minutes. Then set aside to let it cool.

Zest 1 lemon and juice all of the lemons in a bowl. Add the eggs, ¾ cup of erythritol, ¾ cup of almond flour, and salt. Stir together to create the filling. Pour it on top of the cake and cook for 25 minutes. Cut into small pieces and serve with lemon slices.

Nutrition:

Carbohydrates: 4 g

Fat: 26 g

Protein: 8 g

Calories: 272

Creamy Hot Chocolate

Preparation Time: 5 minutes

Cooking time: 5 minutes

Servings: 4

Ingredients:

6 oz dark chocolate, chopped

½ cup unsweetened almond milk

½ cup heavy cream

1 Tbsp erythritol

½ tsp vanilla extract

Directions:

Combine the almond milk, erythritol, and cream in a small saucepan. Heat it (choose medium heat and cook for 1-2 minutes).

Add vanilla extract and chocolate. Stir continuously until the chocolate melts.

Pour into cups and serve.

Nutrition:

Carbohydrates: 4 g

Fat: 18 g

Protein: 2 g

Calories: 193

Delicious Coffee Ice Cream

Preparation Time: 10 minutes

Cooking time: 5 minutes

Servings: 1

Ingredients:

6 ounces coconut cream, frozen into ice cubes

1 ripe avocado, diced and frozen

½ cup coffee expresso

2 Tbsp sweetener

1 tsp vanilla extract

1 Tbsp water

Coffee beans

Directions:

Take out the frozen coconut cubes and avocado from the fridge. Slightly melt them for 5-10 minutes.

Add the sweetener, coffee expresso, and vanilla extract to the coconut-avocado mix and whisk with an immersion blender until it becomes creamy (for about 1 minute). Pour in the water and blend for 30 seconds.

Top with coffee beans and enjoy!

Nutrition:

Carbohydrates: 20.5 g

Fat: 61 g

Protein: 6.3 g

Calories: 596

Fatty Bombs with Cinnamon and Cardamom

Preparation Time: 10 minutes

Cooking time: 35 minutes

Servings: 10

Ingredients:

½ cup unsweetened coconut, shredded

3 oz unsalted butter

¼ tsp ground green cinnamon

¼ ground cardamom

½ tsp vanilla extract

Directions:

Roast the unsweetened coconut (choose medium-high heat) until it begins to turn lightly brown.

Combine the room-temperature butter, half of the shredded coconut, cinnamon, cardamom, and vanilla extract in a separate dish. Cool the mix in the fridge for about 5-10 minutes.

Form small balls and cover them with the remaining shredded coconut.

Cool the balls in the fridge for about 10-15 minutes.

Nutrition:

Carbohydrates: 0.4 g

Fat: 10 g

Protein: 0.4 g

Calories: 90

Raspberry Mousse

Preparation Time: 10 minutes

Cooking time: 4 hours

Servings: 8

Ingredients:

3 oz fresh raspberry

2 cups heavy whipping cream

2 oz pecans, chopped

¼ tsp vanilla extract

½ lemon, the zest

Directions:

Pour the whipping cream into the dish and blend until it becomes soft.

Put the lemon zest and vanilla into the dish and mix thoroughly.

Put the raspberries and nuts into the cream mix and stir well.

Cover the dish with plastic wrap and put it in the fridge for 3 hours.

Top with raspberries and serve.

Nutrition:

Carbohydrates: 3 g

Fat: 26 g

Protein: 2 g

Calories: 255

Chocolate Spread with Hazelnuts

Preparation Time: 5 minutes

Cooking time: 5 minutes

Servings: 6

Ingredients:

2 Tbsp cacao powder

5 oz hazelnuts, roasted and without shells

1 oz unsalted butter

¼ cup coconut oil

Directions:

Whisk all the spread ingredients with a blender for as long as you want. Remember, the longer you blend, the smoother your spread.

Nutrition:

Carbohydrates –2 g

Fat: 28 g

Protein: 4 g

Calories: 271

Quick and Simple Brownie

Preparation Time: 20 minutes

Cooking time: 5 minutes

Servings: 2

Ingredients:

3 Tbsp Keto chocolate chips

1 Tbsp unsweetened cacao powder

2 Tbsp salted butter

2¼ Tbsp powdered sugar

Directions:

Combine 2 Tbsp of chocolate chips and butter, melt them in a microwave for 10-15 minutes. Add the remaining chocolate chips, stir and make a sauce.

Add the cacao powder and powdered sugar to the sauce and whisk well until you have a dough.

Place the dough on a baking sheet, form the Brownie.

Put your Brownie into the oven (preheated to 350°F).

Bake for 5 minutes.

Nutrition:

Carbohydrates: 9 g

Fat: 30 g

Protein: 13 g

Calories: 100

Cute Peanut Balls

Preparation Time: 20 minutes

Cooking time: 20 minutes

Servings: 18

Ingredients:

1 cup salted peanuts, chopped

1 cup peanut butter

1 cup powdered sweetener

8 oz keto chocolate chips

Directions:

Combine the chopped peanuts, peanut butter, and sweetener in a separate dish. Stir well and make a dough. Divide it into 18 pieces and form small balls. Put them in the fridge for 10-15 minutes.

Use a microwave to melt your chocolate chips.

Plunge each ball into the melted chocolate.

Return your balls in the fridge. Cool for about 20 minutes.

Nutrition:

Carbohydrates: 7 g

Fat: 17 g

Protein: 7 g

Calories: 194

Chocolate Mug Muffins

Preparation Time: 5 minutes

Cooking time: 2 minutes

Servings: 4

Ingredients:

4 Tbsp almond flour

1 tsp baking powder

4 Tbsp granulated erythritol

2 Tbsp cocoa powder

½ tsp vanilla extract

2 pinches salt

2 eggs beaten

3 Tbsp butter, melted

1 tsp coconut oil, for greasing the mug

½ oz sugar-free dark chocolate, chopped

Directions:

Mix the dry ingredients together in a separate bowl. Add the melted butter, beaten eggs, and chocolate to the bowl. Stir thoroughly.

Divide your dough into 4 pieces. Put these pieces in the greased mugs and put them in the microwave. Cook for 1-1.5 minutes (700 watts).

Let them cool for 1 minute and serve.

Nutrition:

Carbohydrates: 2 g

Fat: 19 g

Protein: 5 g

Calories: 208

CHAPTER 12:

28-Day Keto Meal Plan for People Over 50

In this chapter, I will give you a 28-day keto meal plan, so you know exactly what you need to eat for each day.

DAYS	BREAKFAST	MAIN MEAL	DESSERT
1.	French omelet	Keto baked salmon with lemon and butter	Sugar-free lemon bars
2.	Sage sausage patty	Ketogenic spicy oyster	Creamy hot chocolate
3.	Feta frittata	Garlic lime mahi-mahi	Delicious coffee ice cream
4.	Ham steak with bacon, mushrooms, and gruyere	Fish and leek sauté	Fatty bombs with cinnamon and cardamom
5.	Mushroom-mascarpone frittata	Smoked salmon salad	Raspberry mousse
6.	Broccoli quiche cups	Keto baked salmon with pesto	Chocolate spread with hazelnuts
7.	Savory chicken sausage-apple	Roasted salmon with parmesan dill crust	Quick and simple brownie
8.	Manchego and shiitake scramble	Keto fried salmon with broccoli and cheese	Cute peanut balls

9.	Three-cheese quiche	Chapter .	Chocolate mug muffins
10.	Breakfast turkey sausage	Herbed beef tenderloin	Sugar-free lemon bars
11.	No-bread breakfast sandwich	Steak with cheese sauce	Creamy hot chocolate
12.	Baked eggs	Steak with pesto	Delicious coffee ice cream
13.	Cured salmon with chives and scrambled eggs	Herbed lamb chops	Fatty bombs with cinnamon and cardamom
14.	Eggs benedict on avocados	Stuffed leg of lamb	Raspberry mousse
15.	French omelet	Grilled pork chops	Chocolate spread with hazelnuts
16.	Sage sausage patty	Pork chops in cream sauce	Quick and simple brownie
17.	Feta frittata	Sweet & tangy pork tenderloin	Cute peanut balls
18.	Ham steak with bacon, mushrooms, and gruyere	Grilled whole chicken	Chocolate mug muffins
19.	Mushroom-mascarpone frittata	Grilled chicken breast	Sugar-free lemon bars
20.	Broccoli quiche cups	Glazed chicken thighs	Creamy hot chocolate
21.	Savory chicken sausage-apple	Bacon-wrapped chicken breasts	Delicious coffee ice cream

22.	Manchego and shiitake scramble	Chicken parmigiana	Fatty bombs with cinnamon and cardamom
23.	Three-cheese quiche	Roasted turkey	Raspberry mousse
24.	Breakfast turkey sausage	Roasted turkey breast	Chocolate spread with hazelnuts
25.	No-bread breakfast sandwich		Quick and simple brownie
26.	Baked eggs	Keto baked salmon with lemon and butter	Cute peanut balls
27.	Cured salmon with chives and scrambled eggs	Ketogenic spicy oyster	Chocolate mug muffins
28.	Eggs benedict on avocados	Garlic lime mahi-mahi	Sugar-free lemon bars

Keep in mind that this meal plan is not for everyone because of allergies or other medical complications, so at least consult your doctor and see what food you cannot eat and customize accordingly. So long as you know how much carbs, fat, and protein you need to consume, you are good to go.

CHAPTER 13:

Common Mistakes In The Ketogenic Diet You Need To Know

Let's now introduce the concept of ketosis: Ketosis is a condition in which the body obtains energy by burning fat and producing so-called ketones. Typically, this situation occurs when blood glucose levels rise due to a decrease in insulin. Low ketosis levels are normal, but when ketones increase a lot in a short time, they can also have serious negative effects.

That is, ketosis is the condition that we must achieve, it is our final result, the reason why we started the ketogenic diet. Knowing this new concept, let's see what the main errors in the ketogenic diet are.

Give up before completing ketosis

Nutritional ketosis is a mandatory step and brings with it more or less evident and more or less long aftermath. This is based on how much carbohydrate has been abused previously and how much our liver is overloaded.

While the body is moving from burning sugar to burning fat, we have the sensation of feeling "poisoned" and "weighed down".

They are the toxins that are rising and, time a week or two, it starts to bloom again.

Other symptoms related to the ketosis that is taking place are:

Bad breath

Slight nausea

An initial hunger for sugars

Tiredness

Nervousness

A slight sadness

These latter symptoms are linked to the impact that the elimination of sugars and carbohydrates has on our mind which, by stimulating the same opiate receptors, make us feel happy and satisfied.

Now by stopping them and losing this stimulus, it may happen that, on the contrary, we feel a little sad and nervous.

Many are frightened of these symptoms and not being well informed, they believe that the ketogenic diet is not for them, that they are worse than when they started and abandon everything before going all the way to ketosis.

Running into deficiencies in salts and minerals

The desire for sugars that is accused at the beginning can be exacerbated by a possible lack of minerals. It is therefore necessary to integrate with the right doses of potassium, magnesium and sodium. Using Himalayan salt, eating salty snacks, using magnesium in the evening, could be just as many ways to remedy this mistake.

Consume too much protein

In the beginning, higher doses of protein help to overcome hunger crises, but then it is good to go back to consuming the right amount. To find out how many proteins to consume, just multiply your body weight by 0.8 (if you make a normal physical effort) or 1.2 (if you are a sportsman).

Another common mistake is to consume poor-quality proteins, such as pork and cold cuts.

Insufficient fat consumption

This is another mistake that is easy to run into in the ketogenic diet. We continue to be afraid of consuming fats and not using all-natural sources: coconut oil, ghee, MCT oil, egg yolk, fatty fish, butter, avocado. The opposite mistake is to exaggerate with oilseeds: walnuts, almonds, flax seeds, pumpkin seeds which, if we neglect to soak in advance with water and lemon, we also absorb the phytic acid they contain, a pro substance inflammatory and antinutrient.

Consume bad quality food

It is another of the most common mistakes. We focus on weight loss, but continue to consume frozen, canned, highly processed food and, as mentioned, proteins that are practical and quick to eat but of poor quality.

Do not introduce the right amount of fiber

Vegetables should always be fresh, consumed in twice the amount of protein and always cooked intelligently, that is, never subjected to overcooking or too high temperatures.

In everyday life, if present, however, we often resort to ready-made, frozen or packaged vegetables.

Also, with regard to fruit, we often resort to the very sugary one, we forget that there are many berries with a low glycemic index: berries, mulberries, goji berries, Inca berries, maqui.

Eat raw vegetables

I know this may surprise you, but consuming large quantities of raw vegetables, centrifuged, cold smoothies, over time slow down digestion, cool it, undermine our ability to transform food and absorb nutrients.

Over time, this exposes us to inevitable deficiencies: joint pain, teeth, nails and weak hair, anemia, tiredness, abnormal weight loss.

Consume the highest protein load at dinner

This is a mistake that involuntarily we all commit. Our job may lead us to stay out all day, to eat a frugal meal for lunch or even not to consume it at all.

Here the dinner turns into the only moment of the day in which we find our family members, we have more time, we are more relaxed and we finally allow ourselves a real meal complete with vegetables, proteins, sometimes even carbohydrates and then fruit or dessert to finish.

During the night, this being busy helping digestion, it cannot perform the other precious task: to purify the blood, prepare hormones, energy for the next day.

Not drinking enough

The number one mistake is don't drink hot water. You got it right, drinking hot water is another story entirely, a huge difference from drinking it even at room temperature.

The benefits are many: greater digestibility and absorption, deep hydration of cells, brighter skin and hair, retention disappears, cellulite improves, kidneys are strengthened, digestion improves, heartburn subsides.

So, in conclusion you have to avoid these nine mistakes:

- Give up before completing ketosis
- Incurring deficiencies in salts and minerals
- Consuming too much protein
- Consume few fats
- Consume bad quality food
- Do not introduce the right amount of fiber
- Consume raw vegetables
- Introduce the highest protein load in the evening
- Do not drink especially hot water

That is, to give the body the opportunity to enter and exit the state of ketosis, to use fats as energy fuel, but also to burn glucose when we have it available.

Benefits of The Keto Diet for People Over 50

So, what exactly can you look forward to once you go on a Ketogenic Diet? There are tons of benefits! Here are some of the pros of this brand-new diet:

Efficient Way to Lose Weight

Let's forget calories for a few minutes and just concentrate on the kind of nutrients you have in your food. A study published in PubMed which allows for a meta-analysis of a randomized controlled trial between a very-low-carbohydrate ketogenic diet versus a low-fat diet for long-term weight loss shows that the low-carb option provides for better long-term results. It can even help reduce risk factors of cardiovascular problems, which simply means that you'll have fewer chances of suffering from heart problems or high blood pressure. The science behind this isn't that complicated. The fact is that the body finds it easier to turn sugar into energy: which is why when given a choice, your body will always choose to run on sugar. Fat is also a possible source of energy – but it takes more work, which is why you lose weight more consistently with a Ketogenic Diet.

Reduces the Risk of Acne

You'd think a person in their 50's wouldn't have acne – and you'd probably be right. Note though that a large part of what you eat affects skin health, even if you're already in your 50s. In fact, people in their 50s need to be extra careful with skin health because this is when growths, blackheads, pore blockages, and more become persistent. Studies show that rapid changes in blood sugar have an effect on skin health as discussed in a study titled: Nutrition and acne – the therapeutic potential of ketogenic diets.

May Help Reduce Cancer Risks

Switching to the Ketogenic Diet may help reduce the risk of cancer, especially as the risk of it increases upon reaching the age of 50. Although that's just a small percentage, it's definitely worth noting – especially if you happen to have a history of cancer in the family. It's also interesting to note that the Ketogenic Diet is usually prescribed as a complement to chemotherapy. A study titled "Ketogenic diets as an adjuvant cancer therapy: history and potential mechanism" concluded that the deprivation of sugar causes more stress to the cancer cells. This simply means that cancer cells depend more on the glucose you have on your body and once their energy source is cut-off, they're more likely to die off.

Reduces Risk of Heart Problems

The healthy fat found in avocado, nuts, and other food items promoted by the Ketogenic Diet can help reduce the possibility of heart problems. In a study titled: The long-term effects of a ketogenic diet in obese patients, it was seen that going on a Keto Diet significantly increases HDL and lowers LDL. HDL is known as the "good cholesterol" while LDL is the "bad cholesterol" known for increasing the likelihood of heart problems. The bad type is still discouraged and is not part of the Ketogenic Diet.

Protects Brain Function

Have you ever found yourself trying to remember simple things – like what things to buy from the store or what day to pay the power bill? Forgetfulness becomes more common as you grow older – but it doesn't have to be! In a study titled: The effects of Ketogenic Diet on behavior and cognition, it was revealed that children following the diet have better cognitive functioning and alertness. It's also theorized that the diet has neurological protective benefits – which basically means that it can help prevent problems that affect brain function. For example, you'll have slightly lower risks of Parkinson's, Alzheimer's, and other forms of dementia.

Bone Health

Osteoporosis becomes more likely as a person advances in age. This is especially true if you weren't able to introduce appropriate amounts of calcium in your body. As you probably know, osteoporosis makes the bone brittle and fragile. This means that your likelihood of having a serious injury from seemingly small accidents increases. A simple slip and bones can fracture or hips may become dislocated. Persistent inflammation of the joints could become an everyday problem. The Ketogenic Diet is a good way of preventing these from happening because the diet naturally involves the intake of healthy dairy or milk products. More importantly, the Ketogenic Diet promotes the intake of low-toxin food products. Hence, your body absorbs food nutrients better, ensuring that all the minerals you need are distributed evenly throughout the body.

But I'm Over 50!

I understand that you have several concerns when using the Ketogenic Diet. Sure, the benefits are definitely great – but many of these benefits are experienced by those who are in their 40s or younger. This means that aside from the excess weight, they don't really have any other health problems to contend with. But what if you're already in your 50s or more? From what I see, most people in their 50s already have several health issues. Usually, these are health problems that occur simply because of age – so don't feel too bad about yourself!

For example, high blood pressure, heart problems, and diabetes are common problems for people in their 50s. If you happen to be in this situation – it's important to first consult your doctor before going on the Ketogenic Diet – or any other diet for that matter. Since we're doing our best to cover all areas of Ketogenic Diet for people over 50, this book will also talk about some of the downsides if you have existing health problems. As someone who has done extensive research and has a ton of personal experiences from working with clients, I want you to know that there is absolutely NOTHING to be afraid of when switching to this brand new dietary plan.

Keto Side Effects and How to Salve Them

It would be very irresponsible of me if I only tell you all the good things about the Ketogenic Diet and ignore the side effects. The truth is that there are negative effects that could happen once you start the Ketogenic Diet – but that's actually true for all of them! All types of diet have negative effects to start with because your body has gotten used to bad habits. Once you make the shift to a more positive way of eating, the body sort of goes on a rebellious phase so it feels like everything is going wrong. For example, a person who used to eat lots of sugar in a day can have severe headaches once they start to avoid sugar. This is a withdrawal symptom and tells you that your diet is actually making positive changes to the body – albeit it takes a little bit of pain on your part.

So what can one expect when they make that change towards a healthy Ketogenic Diet? Here are some of the things to expect and of course – how to troubleshoot these problems.

Long Term Side Effects

A study titled "Metabolic Effects of the Very Low Carbohydrate Diets: Misunderstood Villains of Human Metabolism" shows that for short-term purposes, the Ketogenic Diet is very effective. It lets you burn all those excess fat quickly but in a healthy way. If you do this for a long period of time however, there will be side effects. For example, there can be muscle loss, dizziness, kidney problems, acidosis, and problems with focus. Does that mean you shouldn't go on a Ketogenic Diet at all? Of course not! This only means that you'll have to be careful when using this diet. Don't push it too hard and you will be able to get all the positive results with none of the downsides!

Do you know why a low carbohydrate diet is bad if done for a long time? Well, balance is important in anything you do and the Ketogenic Diet doesn't really support balance. If you get rid of an entire food group for a long period of time, your body will rebel against you. Remember – the Ketogenic Diet relies on stored fat in your body. If there is no more stored fat, it really won't work anymore so you will have to increase your carbohydrates. To solve this problem, I recommend going on a 30-day Ketogenic Diet first and assessing your health before moving forward. Asking your doctor what to do "next" after the 30-day plan or after hitting your weight goal is also a good idea. Personally, I decided to increase my carbohydrate intake slightly after hitting my goal weight.

Keto Flu

The Keto Flu is the most prominent problem you'll encounter when starting the diet. It's a perfectly normal reaction by the body that may seem alarming because, well, the symptoms don't really feel good. You have to understand, your body has been running on a specific type of gasoline for years. It's been taking fuel from sugar and with the Ketogenic Diet, it's like you're changing your fuel source to a cleaner and more sustainable type. It makes sense that the engine growls a little in protest – but after that, you'll be able to run beautifully without the guilt.

The Keto Flu has the following symptoms:

Headaches

Fatigue

Irritability

Brain fog or difficulty focusing

Motivational problems

Sugar cravings

Dizziness

Nausea

Muscle cramps

Frequent urination

These symptoms are all heavily dependent on the kind of person doing the Keto Diet. Since you're already in our 50s, the symptoms may be more prominent, especially if you rely heavily on carbohydrates in your diet. If you eat mostly low-carb food however, these effects may not be as obvious.

But how do you solve them? Here are some of the best ways to get rid of the Keto-Flu as quickly as possible!

First, increase your water and salt consumption. This happens a lot once you start a Ketogenic Diet. You may not notice it, but a lot of the salt you consume is through carbohydrates like bread, pasta, rice, and so on. Salt tends to make you thirsty so if you eat little salt, you're also less likely to look for water during the day. So what happens now? Every time you feel dizzy or tired or nauseous while on a Keto Diet, just dissolve salt in water and gulp it down. Now, this is not going to taste good - but I promise that it will help you feel better. You can always try consuming the salt and water separately – whatever you find most convenient. As for water, try to hit a target of 3 liters of water every day. The good news is that this doesn't have to be plain water – your smoothies, coffee, and tea drinks are also counted.

Add more fat to your diet. Because of all the wrong information circulating today, a lot of people are afraid of fat. We've discussed this before but it bears repeating – fat is not your enemy. During the Ketogenic Diet, it makes sense to eat lots of fats especially if your carbohydrate intake dips to an all-time low. If you lower the carbohydrate consumption without an equal fat increase, then you will always feel hungry and tired.

Conclusion

Routines are very important on this diet, and it's something that will help you stay healthy. As such, in this part, we are going to be giving you tips and tricks to make this diet work better for you and help you get an idea of routines that you can put in place for yourself.

Tip number one that is so important is "drink water!" This is absolutely vital for any diet that you're on, and you need it if not on one as well. However, this vital tip is crucial on a keto diet because when you are eating fewer carbs, you are storing less water, meaning that you are going to get dehydrated very easily. You should aim for more than the daily amount of water; however, remember that drinking too much water can be fatal as your kidneys can only handle so much at once. While this has mostly happened to soldiers in the military, it does happen to dieters as well, so it is something to be aware of.

Along with that same tip is to keep your electrolytes. You have three major electrolytes in your body. When you are on a keto diet, your body is reducing the amount of water that you store. It can be flushing out the electrolytes that your body needs as well, and this can make you sick. Some of the ways that you can battle this is by either salting your food or drinking bone broth. You can also eat pickled vegetables.

Eat when you're hungry instead of snacking or eating constantly. This is also going to help, and when you focus on natural foods and healthy foods, this will help you even more. Eating foods that are processed is the worst thing you can do for fighting cravings, so you should really get into the routine of trying to eat whole foods instead.

Another routine that you can get into is setting a note somewhere that you can see it that will remind you of why you're doing this in the first place and why it's important to you. Dieting is hard, and you will have moments of weakness where you're wondering why you are doing this. Having a reminder will help you feel better, and it can really help with your perspective.

You should make it a daily or everyday routine to try and lower your stress. Stress will not allow you to get into ketosis, which is that state that keto wants to put you in. The reason for this being that stress increases the hormone known as cortisol in your blood, and it will prevent your body from being able to burn fats for energy. This is because your body has too much sugar in your blood. If you're going through a really high period of stress right now in your life, then this diet is not a great idea. Some great ideas for this would be getting into the habit or routine of taking the time to do something relaxing, like walking and making sure that you're getting enough sleep, leads to the following routine that you need to do.

You need to get enough sleep. This is so important not just for your diet but also for your mind and body as well. Poor sleep also raises those stress hormones that can cause issues for you, so you need to get into the routine of getting seven hours of sleep at night on the minimum and nine hours if you can. If you're getting less than this, you need to change the routine you have in place right now and make sure that you establish a new routine where you are getting more sleep. As a result, your health and diet will be better.

www.ingramcontent.com/pod-product-compliance
Lightning Source LLC
Chambersburg PA
CBHW081417080526
44589CB00016B/2570